Acupuncture: a scientific appraisal

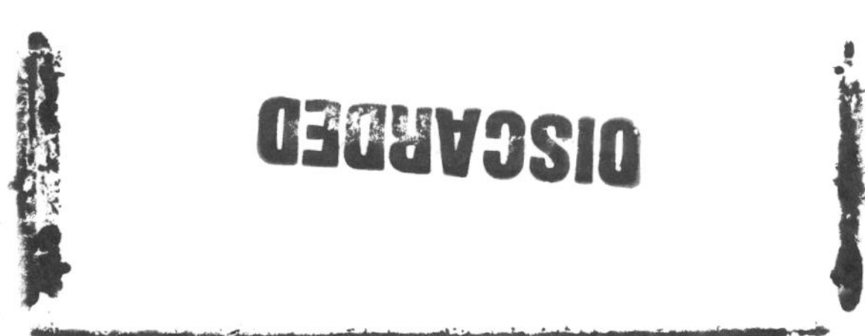

Acupuncture: a scientific appraisal

Edited by

Professor Edzard Ernst MD PhD FRCP
Director
Department of Complementary Medicine
School of Postgraduate Medicine and Health Sciences
University of Exeter
UK

and

Dr Adrian White MA BM BCh
Research Fellow
Department of Complementary Medicine
School of Postgraduate Medicine and Health Sciences
University of Exeter
UK

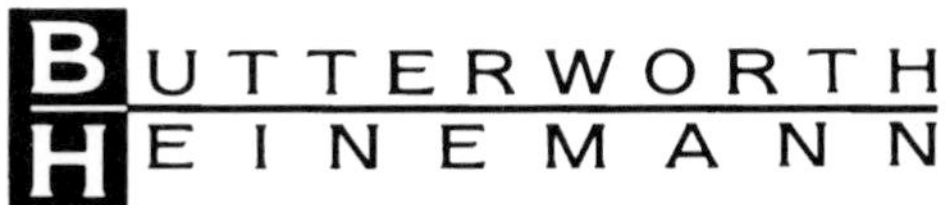

OXFORD AUCKLAND BOSTON JOHANNESBURG MELBOURNE NEW DELHI

Butterworth-Heinemann
Linacre House, Jordan Hill, Oxford OX2 8DP
225 Wildwood Avenue, Woburn, MA 01801-2041
A division of Reed Educational and Professional Publishing Ltd

A member of the Reed Elsevier plc Group

First published 1999
Reprinted 2000

British Library Cataloguing in Publication Data
A catalogue copy of this book is available from the British Library

Library of Congress Cataloguing in Publication Data
A catalogue copy of this book is available from the Library of Congress

ISBN 0 7506 4163 0

Typeset by E & M Graphics, Midsomer Norton, Bath
Printed and bound by MPG Books Ltd, Bodmin, Cornwall

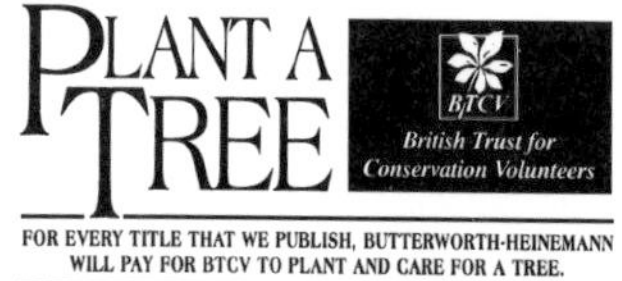

Contents

Contributors

Stephen Birch
Founding Member, Society for Acupuncture Research; Acupuncturist, The Netherlands

Michael Cummings
Director of Education, British Medical Acupuncture Society, UK

Edzard Ernst
Director, Department of Complementary Medicine, School of Postgraduate Medicine and Health Sciences, University of Exeter, UK

Jacqueline Filshie
Consultant Anaesthetist, The Royal Marsden NHS Trust, Sutton, Surrey; Honorary Senior Lecturer, Institute of Cancer Research, Sutton, Surrey, UK

Ted Kaptchuk
Assistant Professor of Medicine, Harvard Medical School; Associate Director, Centre for Alternative Medical Research and Education, Beth Israel Deaconess Medical School, Boston, Massachusetts, USA

Thomas Lundeberg
Head, Section of Integrative Sensory Physiology, Karolinska Institute; Chief of Medical Services, Section of Alternative Medicine, Karolinska Hospital, Stockholm, Sweden

Elmar Peuker
Institute of Anatomy, Westphalian Wilhelms-University, Muenster, Germany

Hagen Rampes
Consultant Psychiatrist, Ealing, Hammersmith and Fulham Mental Health NHS Trust, Southall, Middlesex, UK

Adrian White
Research Fellow, Department of Complementary Medicine, School of Postgraduate Medicine and Health Sciences, University of Exeter, UK

Introduction

Adrian White and Edzard Ernst

A fifth-century anecdote from China tells how Zhen Quan cured the shoulder problem of the governor of the province of Lu Zhou. The problem was severe and interfered with his archery. The celebrated physician Zhen Quan was summoned. He told the governor to turn to face the target with his bow and arrow and take aim. As he did so, Zhen Quan stood behind him and, taking advantage of the raised arm, thrust a needle in the acupuncture point known as Jian-Yu, on the tip of the shoulder. The response was immediate: the arrow flew straight to the centre of the target. Zhen Quan's eminent reputation was confirmed (Ma, 1992).

The history of acupuncture is loaded with anecdotes. The purpose of this book is to look for evidence: how did Zhen Quan know which point to use? Did the governor recover through a specific effect of the needle, through the power of Zhen Quan's reputation, or was it a spontaneous remission or natural regression? If it was the acupuncture, what mechanisms were involved? What was Zhen Quan's success rate with other conditions? What side-effects did the governor risk?

What is acupuncture?

The term 'acupuncture' is used in this book to refer to the insertion of dry needles into the body, at specially chosen sites, for the treatment or prevention of symptoms and conditions. Acupressure and other methods of non-needle stimulation (such as moxibustion, TENS) are not generally covered in this text.

There are a large number of variations in acupuncture practice, ranging between two typical approaches. On the one hand, a practitioner of traditional Chinese medicine will make an individual diagnosis in 'energetic' terms by interpreting the patient's symptoms and signs according to certain theories. He or she will place needles in recognized acupuncture points, is likely to stimulate them for a minute or so by manipulation, and then leave them for about 20 minutes while the patient is resting. The acupuncturist may also issue a prescription for Chinese herbs, give lifestyle advice and dietary recommendations. On the other hand, a western-style acupuncturist will use a conventional history and examination to make an orthodox diagnosis and will regard acupuncture as one of a range of therapeutic options. He or she will believe that the needles stimulate nerve endings and will choose points with that purpose. Needling may be quite brief and involve different strengths of stimulation. There is no reason to exclude either approach from our scientific appraisal.

Brief history of acupuncture

The origins of acupuncture are lost in Chinese prehistory and rooted in the mythology of ancient China and Taoist thinking. The oldest known text is the Yellow Emperor's *Classic of Internal Medicine* (*Huang Ti Nei Ching*), which probably accumulated over several centuries up to the definitive version of about the first century BC. The *Classic of Internal Medicine* covered all forms of medicine, including moxibustion, acupuncture and herbs. The Yellow Emperor himself lived around 2600 BC, and the work was dedicated to him as a tribute to his excellence. A period of development of acupuncture by observation and teaching from experience followed. By the time of a second systematic description in *The Classic of Acupuncture* (*Zhen Jiu Jia Jing*), about 259 AD, the names and reputed functions of all the points were established (Ma, 1992).

Acupuncture continued to flourish in China, especially throughout the period of the Ming dynasty of 1368–1644. After that, it went into gradual decline, and came to be regarded as 'an insignificant and petty skill'. In 1822 the Emperor Dao Guang banned acupuncture and moxibustion from the Forbidden City on the grounds that they were not suitable forms of treatments for a monarch. In the early part of the twentieth century acupuncture's popularity among the Chinese waxed and waned as opposing factions in society held sway, one wanting to rid China of everything superstitious and unscientific, their opponents not wanting to surrender Chinese culture to western influence. As western medicine was introduced it was regarded as superior and traditional medicine was relegated to rural areas and no longer taught in the medical schools (Ma, 1992).

Acupuncture was reintroduced by the Communist government in the 1950s for pragmatic reasons: the urgent need for some sort of provision of some sort of medical services to the population of half a billion people (Bonica, 1974). Barefoot doctors were given crash courses in acupuncture and herbal medicine. Chairman Mao taught: 'Chinese medicine and pharmacology are a great treasure-house, and efforts should be made to explore them and raise them to a higher level' (Peking Children's Hospital, 1975). Acupuncture soon became re-established, so that today in China, western and traditional treatment are often offered side by side.

Acupuncture gradually spread to the rest of the world over the course of several centuries. In 552 AD acupuncture was presented to the Japanese court and increased in popularity there over the next 200 years (Ma, 1992). Reports of acupuncture were first brought back to the west by Jesuit missionaries in the sixteenth century. A more accurate description was given in 1683 by Dr Willen Ten Rhijne, a physician working for the

Dutch East Indies Company in Nagasaki, Japan (Baldry, 1993). Acupuncture was practised widely by French physicians by the late nineteenth century, and the scholar-diplomat Soulier DeMorant published an influential treatise on the subject (Kaplan, 1997). In the USA, acupuncture was known to Osler and mentioned in his textbook *The Principles and Practice of Medicine* (1912): 'For lumbago, acupuncture is, in acute cases, the most efficient treatment'. However, in later editions of the textbook all reference to acupuncture was deleted (Ulett, 1996).

A great surge of interest in acupuncture followed President Nixon's visit to China in 1971. A member of the president's press corps, the *New York Times* reporter James Reston, developed appendicitis. He was given acupuncture for postoperative pain relief, and wrote a graphic account of his experiences for his avid readers (Kaplan, 1997). American physicians visiting China during subsequent years saw surgery being performed with apparently only acupuncture needles for anaesthetic, and the interest of the public and the research community was fired.

Public usage of acupuncture in the West

The prevalence of acupuncture in various countries has been estimated by several surveys, as shown in Table A.

The wide variation, for example from 21% in France to 1% in the USA, probably reflects differences in national regulations affecting the availability of acupuncture. Most likely, it is also due to differences in the survey methodology, including poor response rates and the use of non-random samples, such as readers of a particular newspaper. Telephone surveys of random population samples are undoubtedly more rigorous, and those of a Gallup Poll (Gallup, 1986), Eisenberg *et al.* (1993), MacLennan *et al.* (1996) and Landmark Healthcare (1998) give the most reliable figures. Approximately 1–2% of a typical western population visits an acupuncturist each year. Over a lifetime, this figure rises to about 4% of the population.

Table A Public use of acupuncture, by country

Country	*Author and year*	*Used in last 12 months (%)*	*Ever used (%)*
Belgium	quoted in Fisher and Ward, 1994		19
Denmark	quoted in Fisher and Ward, 1994		12
France	quoted in Fisher and Ward, 1994		21
Netherlands	quoted in Fisher and Ward, 1994		16
Scotland	Emslie *et al.*, 1996		6
Sweden	quoted in Fisher and Ward, 1994		12
UK	quoted in Fisher and Ward, 1994		16
UK	Gallup, 1986		3
USA	quoted in Fisher and Ward, 1994		3
USA	Eisenberg *et al.*, 1993	1	
Australia	MacLennan *et al.*, 1996	2	
USA	Landmark Healthcare, 1998	2	

The prevalence of acupuncture among certain subgroups of the population can be considerably higher: for example, Vecchio (1994) found that 21 out of 280 patients (7.5%) attending a rheumatological outpatients' clinic in Australia had received acupuncture in the past, 20 of them in the previous 12 months. Also, acupuncture was among the commonest therapies used by AIDS patients (Ernst, 1997)

Attitudes of the public

There seems to be an increasing acceptance of complementary medicine in general. Acupuncture is among the best known and most accepted of all complementary therapies (MORI, 1989). A random survey of the public in Scotland found that 94% of respondents knew about acupuncture (Emslie *et al.*, 1996). Moreover, 25% would consider using it, a percentage only exceeded by manipulation; and 54% believed that it should be publicly funded, the highest figure for any complementary therapy. By contrast, only 6% had actually used acupuncture in the past (compared with 14% who had used manipulation).

Attitudes of the medical profession

Among UK medical students, Rampes *et al.* (1997) found that acupuncture was the complementary therapy of most interest. More than 80% would have liked instruction in the principles of acupuncture during their undergraduate training, and 50% would have liked instruction in the practice of acupuncture.

Since 1990, several surveys have been conducted among doctors,

Table B Physicians' willingness to endorse or refer patients for acupuncture treatment, and their belief in its validity

Country	*Author and year*	*Endorse therapy or refer patients (%)*	*Belief (%)*	*Belief question asked*
Canada	Verhoef and Sutherland, 1995		58	belief in efficacy
Netherlands	Knipschild *et al.*, 1990		50	belief in efficacy
Norway	Aasland *et al.*, 1997		46	belief in efficacy
Sweden	Lynoe and Svensson, 1992		23	positive attitude
UK	Anderson and Anderson, 1987	20	15	valid theoretical basis
UK	Perkin *et al.*, 1994	66		none
UK	Thomas *et al.*, 1995	22		none
UK	Wharton and Lewith, 1986		16	useful
UK	White *et al.*, 1997	29	65	belief in efficacy
USA	Berman *et al.*, 1995	23	56	legitimate medical practice
USA	Blumberg *et al.*, 1995	56		none

mostly family physicians (primary care practitioners, general practitioners), posing different questions about their belief of acupuncture (Table B). At least a quarter, and usually more than a half, of respondents have a positive attitude or believe that acupuncture works. Doctors' belief in acupuncture is reflected in their widespread willingness to endorse a patient's decision to receive acupuncture, or to refer patients. Between 25 and 50% of physicians are prepared to refer patients (Table B).

Acupuncture is often the most frequently recommended complementary therapy, or second only to manipulation (White *et al.*, 1997). However, in the survey by Berman *et al.* (1995) acupuncture was eighth in the list of alternative therapies to which family physicians referred their patients. Here again we see the impact of national legislation. Thomas *et al.* (1995) assessed the degree of antagonism that doctors held towards complementary medicine: when asked if they would advise their patients against using acupuncture, less than 1% of UK GPs said they would; 11% had a neutral attitude. Antagonism towards acupuncture was lower than towards any other complementary therapy.

Physicians are handicapped in their assessment of acupuncture by the lack of objective information. About 10% of Norwegian doctors (Aasland *et al.*, 1997) and 30% of British GPs (White *et al.*, 1997) rated their knowledge of acupuncture as 'good'. One study (Anderson and Anderson, 1987) found that only 15% of GPs thought acupuncture had a valid theoretical basis. More recently, Verhoef and Sutherland (1995) asked respondents to state on what they based their opinion on the effectiveness of complementary medicine; most said anecdotal evidence.

In the UK, acupuncture is available within 34% of primary care centres (Thomas *et al.*, 1995) and 86% of chronic pain services (Clinical Standards Advisory Group Report, 1999). Acupuncture is also used in 37% of hospices (Wilkes, 1992).

Indications for acupuncture

An acupuncture service in the Faculty Hospital of Brno-Bohunice in the former Czechoslovakia saw 14 340 patients in its first 10 years (Umlauf, 1988). The main indications for treatment were classified as locomotor disorders (65%), allergic diseases (12%), neurological disorders including headache, migraine, trigeminal neuralgia, facial palsy (9%), neuroses and neurovegetative disorders (8%), and 'other diseases without serious structural changes' (6%).

Wadlow and Peringer (1996) conducted a survey of selected practitioners of traditional Chinese medicine in the UK, who were asked to record data from patients treated during a defined period of time. More than two-thirds of the patients were female, and more patients were aged 40–49 than any other decade. (This can be seen to contrast with general medical services in the UK, which are primarily used by the very young and very old.) The most common indications for treatment are given in Table C. Table D lists the eight conditions most commonly treated by medical acupuncturists in the UK (Hayhoe and Box, 1997). Similar results were obtained for US doctors by Diehl *et al.* (1997).

Table C Numbers and percentages of patients with particular conditions treated by 94 traditional-style acupuncturists in the UK (Adapted from Wadlow and Peringer, 1996)

Condition	*No.*	*%*
musculoskeletal: pain, stiffness, trauma	139	19.5
emotional and psychological	65	9.1
arthritis (rheumatoid and osteo-)	50	7.0
ear, nose and throat (ENT) conditions	49	6.9
low energy, including chronic fatigue syndrome	48	6.7
digestive conditions	45	6.3
back pain: acute and chronic	45	6.3
headache, migraine	43	6.0
gynaecological and obstetric	42	5.9
skin conditions	33	4.6
cardiovascular conditions, including stroke	29	4.1
respiratory conditions	27	3.8
neurological conditions, including herpetic neuralgia	25	3.5
smoking cessation	24	3.4

Acupuncturists

Regulations governing practice of acupuncture vary considerably between countries. In many European countries under Napoleonic statute, acupuncture is officially restricted to practice by those who have undergone formal medical training (British Medical Association, 1993). In Australia and the UK, however, the legislation is permissive, so that anyone may use the title acupuncturist. The only restriction in these countries is a requirement that the premises are checked for hygiene standards. In the USA, non-physician acupuncturists are licensed, registered or certified in 34 states; physicians are allowed to practise acupuncture in all states.

In the UK, five organizations had a total of 3834 practitioners registered in 1997 (Mills and Peacock, 1997). The authors estimated that this figure probably represents about half the acupuncturists working in the country. A large proportion of UK doctors and physiotherapists offer acupuncture as part of their NHS treatment (Dale, 1997). In Germany, it is estimated that 20 000 practitioners use acupuncture (E. Peuker,

Table D Numbers and percentages of 178 medical acupuncturists who use acupuncture for the particular conditions (Adapted from Hayhoe and Box, 1997)

Order	*Condition*	*No.*	*%*
1	musculoskeletal	178	100
2	general pain	157	88
3	neurological	104	58
4	allergy	90	51
5	addiction	90	51
6	ENT	79	44
7	respiratory	75	42
8	gynaecological	73	41

personal communication). In the USA in 1997 there were 8729 licensed acupuncturists (J.K. Rotchford, personal communication).

Because acupuncture is indicated for the sort of problems that are usually managed in primary care, one might expect primary care physicians to be interested in practising it. Acupuncture is used by over 4% of UK family practitioners, and is the second most popular complementary therapy in medicine, after homoeopathy (White *et al.*, 1997).

A survey of German doctors found that acupuncture was practised by 15%, lying sixth behind herbal medicine (78%), neural therapy (65%), homoeopathy (45%), dietary therapy (23%) and chiropractic (20%) (Himmel *et al.*, 1993). Table E gives the percentages of primary care physicians practising acupuncture in different countries.

There is a wide range of results, because the samples were not comparable. For example, Blumberg *et al.* (1995) mailed randomly chosen doctors, whereas Berman *et al.* (1995) surveyed doctors attending a conference.

The numbers of doctors who are practising acupuncture appears to be rising: annual membership of the British Medical Acupuncture Society is shown in Figure A. Not every doctor who trains in acupuncture continues to practise it: for example, Berman *et al.* (1995) found that 22% had trained in the therapy, but only 14% had used it in practice.

Integration of acupuncture

There has recently been considerable impetus behind greater integration of complementary medicine within the UK National Health Service (Foundation for Integrated Medicine, 1997). In the USA, a conference organized by the National Institutes of Health published a consensus statement which concluded that there was sufficient evidence of acupuncture's value to expand its use into conventional medicine (NIH, 1997).

Table E Percentages of physicians who practise acupuncture in different countries, in date order

Country	*Author and year*	*Sample*	*% who practise acupuncture*
Scotland	Reilly, 1983	not random	1
New Zealand	Hadley, 1988	population, local	18
England	Wharton and Lewith, 1986	population, local	21
England	Anderson and Anderson, 1987	population, local	3
New Zealand	Marshall *et al.*, 1990	random	21
Sweden	Lynoe and Svensson, 1992	not random	25
Germany	Himmel *et al.*, 1993	random	15
USA	Blumberg *et al.*, 1994	random	1
UK	Thomas *et al.*, 1995	random	5
USA	Berman *et al.*, 1995	not random	14
UK	White *et al.*, 1997	population, local	4

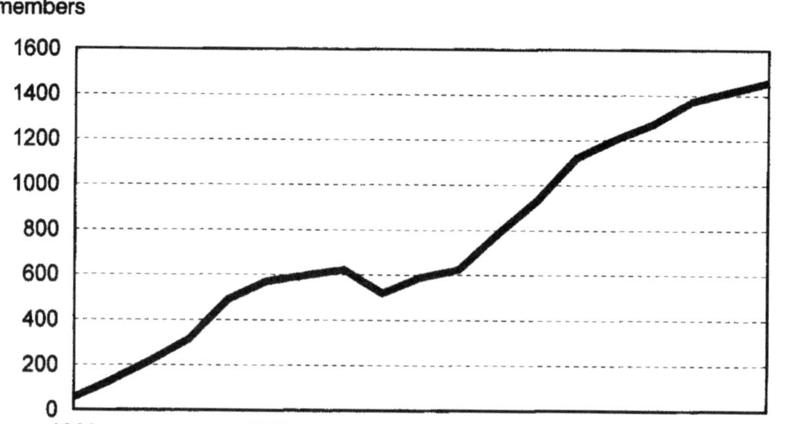

Figure A Growth in membership of the British Medical Acupuncture Society since its foundation in 1980.

Since the development of the concept of evidence-based health care, therapies must establish their efficacy, safety and cost-effectiveness by means of rigorous studies. This is now generally considered to be the best way to provide optimal benefit at minimal risk for patients, and to ensure the equitable use of scarce resources. This book is aimed at summarizing the relevant evidence related to acupuncture in an impartial fashion. It therefore provides a basis for informed decisions.

References

Aasland, O. G., Borchgrevink, C. F. and Fugelli, P. (1997). Complementary medicine – knowledge, attitudes and experiences among Norwegian physicians. *Tidsskr. Nor. Laegeforen.*, **117**, 2464–2468.

Anderson, E. and Anderson, P. (1987). General practitioners and alternative medicine. *J. R. Coll. Gen. Pract.*, **37**, 52–55.

Baldry, P. E. (1993). Acupuncture, trigger points and musculoskeletal pain. Edinburgh: Churchill Livingstone.

Berman, B. M., Singh, B. K., Lao, L. *et al.* (1995). Physicians' attitudes toward complementary or alternative medicine: a regional survey. *J. Am. Board Fam. Pract.*, **8**, 361–366.

Blumberg, D. L., Grant, W. D., Hendricks, S. R. *et al.* (1995). The physician and unconventional medicine. *Alt. Therapies*, **1**(3), 31–35.

British Medical Association (1993). *Complementary Medicine: New Approaches to Good Practice.* Oxford: Oxford University Press.

Bonica, J. J. (1974). Therapeutic acupuncture in the People's Republic of China. *JAMA*, **228,** 1544–1551.

Clinical Standards Advisory Group Report (1999). National Review of Pain Services and Standards. London: The Stationery Office.

Dale, J. (1997). Acupuncture practice in the UK. Part 1: report of a survey. *Comp. Ther. Med.*, **5**, 215–220.

Diehl, D. L., Kaplan, G., Coulter, I. *et al.* (1997). Use of acupuncture by American physicians. *J. Altern. Comp. Med.*, **3**, 119–126.

Eisenberg, D. M., Kessler, R. C., Foster, C. *et al.* (1993). Unconventional medicine in the United States. *New Engl. J. Med.*, **328,** 246–252.

Emslie, M., Campbell, M. and Walker, K. (1996). Complementary therapies in a local healthcare setting. Part 1: Is there a real public demand? *Comp. Ther. Med.*, **4,** 39–42.

Ernst, E. (1997). Complementary AIDS therapies: the good, the bad and the ugly. *Int. J. STD AIDS*, **8,** 281–285.

Fisher, P. and Ward, A. (1994). Complementary medicine in Europe. *Br. Med. J.*, **309,** 107–111.

Foundation for Integrated Medicine (1997). *Integrated Healthcare: A Way Forward for the Next Five Years? A Discussion Document.* Foundation for Integrated Medicine.

Gallup (1986). *Omnibus Report: Alternative Medicine.* Gallup International, 25 Coburn Road, London, E3.

Hadley, C. M. (1988). Complementary medicine and the general practitioner: a survey of general practitioners in the Wellington area. *N. Z. Med. J.*, **101,** 766–768.

Hayhoe, S. and Box, H. (1997). A questionnaire on medical acupuncture practice. *Acup. Med.*, **15,** 96–99.

Himmel, W., Schulte, M. and Kochen, M. K. (1993). Complementary medicine: are patients' expectations being met by their general practitioners? *Br. J. Gen. Pract.*, **43,** 232–235.

Kaplan, G. (1997). A brief history of acupuncture's journey to the West. *J. Alt. Comp. Med.*, **3,** 5–10.

Knipschild, P., Kleijnen, J., Ter Riet, K. (1990). Belief in the efficacy of alternative medicine among general practitioners in the Netherlands. *Soc. Sci. Med.*, **31,** 625–626.

Landmark Healthcare (1998). *The Landmark Report on Public Perceptions of Alternative Care.* Michigan: Landmark Healthcare Inc.

Lynoe, N. and Svensson, T. (1992). Physicians and alternative medicine – an investigation of attitudes and practice. *Scand. J. Soc. Med.*, **20,** 55–60.

Ma, K-W. (1992). The roots and development of Chinese acupuncture: from prehistory to early 20th century. *Acupunct. Med.*, **10**(suppl), 92–99.

MacLennan, A. H., Wilson, D. H. and Taylor, A. W. (1996). Prevalence and cost of alternative medicine in Australia. *Lancet*, **347,** 569–573.

Marshall, R. J., Gee, R., Dumble, J. *et al.* (1990). The use of alternative therapies by Auckland general practitioners. *N. Z. Med. J.*, **103,** 213–215.

Mills, S. and Peacock, W. (1997). *Professional Organisation of Complementary and Alternative Medicine in the United Kingdom: A Report to the Department of Health.* Exeter, Devon: Centre for Complementary Health Studies, University of Exeter.

MORI (1989). *Alternative Medicine Survey.* London: MORI.

NIH (1997). Consensus Statement Online 1997. http://odp.od.nih.gov/consensus/statements/cdc/107/107stmt.html Question1.

Peking Children's Hospital (1975). A clinical analysis of 1,474 operations under acupuncture anesthesia among children. *Chin. Med. J.*, **1,** 369–374.

Perkin, M. R., Pearcy, R. M. and Fraser, J. S. (1994). A comparison of the attitudes shown by general practitioners, hospital doctors and medical students towards alternative medicine. *J. R. Soc. Med.*, **87,** 523–525.

Rampes, H., Sharples, F., Maragh, S. and Fisher, P. (1997). Introducing complementary medicine into the medical curriculum. *J. R. Soc. Med.*, **90,** 19–22.

Reilly, D. T. (1983). Young doctors' views on alternative medicine. *Br. Med. J.*, **287,** 337–339.

Thomas, K., Fall, M., Parry, G. and Nicholl, J. (1995). *National Survey of Access to Complementary Health Care via General Practice. DoH Report.* Sheffield: Medical Care Research Unit.

Ulett, G. A. (1996). Conditioned healing with electroacupuncture. *Altern. Ther. Health Med.*, **2,** 56–60.

Umlauf, R. (1988). Analysis of the main results of the activity of the acupuncture department of faculty hospital. *Acupunct. Med.*, **5**(2), 16–18.

Vecchio, P. C. (1994). Attitudes to alternative medicine by rheumatology outpatient attenders. *J. Rheumatol.*, **21,** 145–147.

Verhoef, M. J. and Sutherland, L. R. (1995). General practitioners' assessment of and interest in alternative medicine in Canada. *Soc. Sci. Med.*, **41,** 511–515.

Wadlow, G. and Peringer, E. (1996). Retrospective survey of patients of practitioners of traditional Chinese acupuncture in the UK. *Comp. Ther. Med.*, **4,** 1–7.

Wharton, R. and Lewith, G. (1986). Complementary medicine and the general practitioner. *Br. Med. J.*, **292,** 1498–1500.

White, A. R., Resch, K-L. and Ernst, E. (1997). Complementary medicine: use and attitudes among GPs. *Fam. Pract.*, **14,** 302–306.

Wilkes, E. (1992). *Complementary Therapy in Hospice and Palliative Care. Report for Trent Palliative Care Centre.*

1

History, nature and current practice of acupuncture: an East Asian perspective

Stephen Birch and Ted Kaptchuk

Introduction

Acupuncture in the west has benefited from its exotic and mysterious connections. Unfortunately, the western understanding of acupuncture and East Asian medicine in general has suffered from an obscurist and romantic view that has ignored the complexity and diversity of this long tradition of healing. Fascination with the exotic and unusual aspects has not been well balanced by information and accurate translation of the tradition from various points in its historical development. This chapter will examine the history, nature, current practice of acupuncture, the shared unity of the tradition and explore the often underexamined heterogeneity of the tradition.

History

Acupuncture is generally believed to have originated in China and has an extensive body of literature that began around 200 BCE continuing to the present (see Sivin, 1987: 16; Unschuld, 1990: 1; Xue, 1991; Birch and Tsutani, 1996). It has been practised in a number of Asian countries for centuries, for example, in Japan for over 1450 years, Korea for at least 1500 years, Vietnam for probably 2000 years, arriving in Europe around 300 years ago and North America over 150 years ago (see Lu and Needham, 1980: 69ff, 262ff; Birch and Felt, 1999), and in the last 30 years has spread to most countries around the world (WHO, 1985: 13).

The earliest major documents, the *Huang Di Nei Jing Su Wen*, *Huang Di Nei Jing Ling Shu* (circa 200 BC) and the *Nan Jing* (circa 100 AD), are revered as the primary sources of acupuncture and have been commented on by numerous authors over the centuries (Ishihara, 1983; Unschuld, 1986: 653–669; Sivin, 1987: 24). For many acupuncturists today, these texts are still held in high regard and are often studied. Frequently the authenticity of a particular tradition or practitioner's approach is claimed by citing appropriate passages from these and later historical texts. The validity of many ideas in modern practice is claimed by citing appropriate passages from these historical texts. Many texts use this method (e.g. see Kaptchuk, 1983; Maciocia, 1989; Matsumoto and Birch,

1988; Shudo, 1990; Soulie de Morant, 1994). However much of what the historical texts describe has been unclear for centuries, hence the large number of commentaries on them. Lack of clarity in the literature is a result of many factors, among which are problems in the vagueness of original expression (see e.g. Unschuld's multi-commentated translation of the *Nan Jing* (Unschuld, 1986)), problems in understanding terminology outside the culture in which it arose and was used (see discussions in Porkert, 1974: 1–8; Needham and Lu, 1975; Unschuld, 1989; Wiseman and Boss, 1990; Wiseman, 1995), problems of contradictory statements in the same text (see discussions in Epler (1980)), and problems of disagreement between texts (e.g. see Yanagiya, 1948: 1–38; and discussions in Sivin, 1987: 126–131). These factors, combined with the varying sociopolitical and cultural climates in each of the countries where acupuncture has been practised (e.g. see Kaptchuk, 1985; Unschuld, 1985), have fostered a wide variety of conceptual models for clinical practice and multiple methods and techniques of practice. This variety is now so immense that it is almost misleading to simply call it 'acupuncture'. In terms of techniques used by acupuncturists, not only have needling (acus) and puncturing not always been common to all systems of practice, but there is also a wide range of ancillary techniques routinely used by different systems of practice. Further, the use of a single term is understood by many to imply a coherent and uniform model of practice both in the modern era and from its inception, ideas clearly not in keeping with established historical facts.

Basic terminology and concepts

The term 'acupuncture' is a loose translation of the Chinese term 'zhenjiu' (Japanese 'shinkyu'), which actually means 'zhen' – needle (therapy) – and 'jiu' – cauterization/moxa (therapy). The term acupuncture comes from late seventeenth century Europe and is often used to refer to both 'zhen' and 'jiu', though strictly speaking it refers more to the use of needles, zhen (Lu and Needham, 1980: 1). The practice of jiu has been called moxibustion after the Japanese word 'mogusa', ('moxa') (Porkert, 1974: 40; Lu and Needham, 1980: 291–292), and refers to burning small pieces of punk of the dried *Artemisia vulgaris* (mugwort) plant. Thus when most people speak of acupuncture they are more accurately speaking of acupuncture and moxibustion, or as it has more recently been translated, 'acu–moxa therapy' (e.g. Wiseman and Ellis, 1985).

Much of the historical literature describes both zhen and jiu. However there were specialized texts that described only the practice of zhen, needling (see e.g. the *Nan Jing* (circa 100 CE), perhaps the most important early exclusively acupuncture text; see Unschuld, 1986). There were also specialized texts that described only the practice of jiu, moxibustion (e.g. see the *Zu Bi Shi Yi Mai Jiu Jing* and *Yin Yang Shi Yi Mai Jiu*, both found in the Ma Wang-dui dig dating from circa 200 BCE, the *Ming Tang Jiu Jing* (1126 CE), the *Bei Ji Jiu Fa* (1226 CE), the *Bian Que Xin Shu* (1289 CE) and the *Shen Jiu Jing Lun* (1851 CE)). For discussions of these, see Birch and Felt (1999), Birch and Ida (1998) and Lu and Needham (1980: 176ff). This point is important when we look to modern practice. In China, the acupuncturist is trained in both needle and moxa (acu–moxa) therapy, with the scope of practice covering both. The use of each method is based upon certain principles and a case by case judgement. In Japan, needle and moxa therapies are separately licensed, and, while most acupuncturists learn and practice both, there are 'moxibustionists', specialists who use only moxa, and some acupuncturists who use only needles. The range of medical disorders that practitioners of one or both methods claim to treat is very similar. (For discussions of training, scope of practice and licensure, see Nakagawa, 1987; Sivin, 1987: 441–442; Sonoda, 1988: 78; Ergil 1994; Mitchell, 1996. For examples of diverse acupuncture, moxibustion and acu–moxa therapy literature, see: Ulett (1992) for needling, Irie (1980) for moxibustion, and O'Connor and Bensky (1981) and So (1987) for acu–moxa therapy.) The acupuncture practitioner can generally use a wide variety of other treatment methods and techniques, according to training, school and personal preferences. Hence the practice of acupuncture is generally not restricted to needling.

It is frequently claimed that acupuncture is part of a larger system of practice. In so far as acupuncture is one of the traditional medicines of countries like China, Japan, Korea and Vietnam, then acupuncture can be said to be part of the 'traditional medicine' from those countries. But this does not necessarily imply that it is an integral part of traditional medicine, as is stated by many authors (e.g. see Beinfield and Korngold, 1991; Rosenthal, 1987: 37). We must look to the history of practice of acupuncture to see if it has been a necessary integral part, an independently functioning part, or a sometimes necessary part of the practice of traditional medicine. We must also look to see if there are coherent and continuous models and traditions of practice. In China today, acupuncture is seen as part of the practice of 'zhong yi' or 'Chinese medicine' or 'traditional Chinese medicine, TCM' (for a good discussion of 'zhong yi' see Sivin, 1987: 3, 20ff; Unschuld, 1985: 250ff). This term is said to encompass all traditional forms of medical practice (e.g. see Beinfield and Korngold, 1991), despite the clear documentation of it excluding some forms of traditional medicine (Unschuld, 1985: 250; Sivin, 1987: 23). Zhong yi is thought by many to imply a coherent theory underlying these diverse medical therapies (e.g. see Larre *et al.*, 1986: 27). In particular zhong yi was given a relatively uniform theoretical basis through which acupuncture and moxibustion practices were combined with 'zhong cao yao' or the traditional system of Chinese drugs and herbal medicines (Kaptchuk, 1983: 79–83). These different medical traditions had theoretical bases that appeared somewhat similar, and historically the combined or separate practice of them had always been a matter of personal choice, evidenced by the multitude of texts that described acupuncture, moxibustion, herbal medicine or combinations of these. However, in the 1950s they were placed under one heading primarily to serve the political and public health needs of China after the 1949 liberation (e.g. see Hillier and Jewell, 1983: 66ff). This gave the appearance of a uniform and integrated system of medical practice, which has strongly influenced the dissemination and practice of acupuncture in the west – acupuncture and moxibustion are now commonly practised with herbal therapeutics under a single banner called 'traditional Chinese medicine' (TCM). However, the situation in China is actually more complex with a routine separation in the teaching and practice of acu–moxa therapy and herbal medicine (Ergil, 1993, 1994), and an increasingly more visible re-emergence of varied traditions of practice.

In Japan acupuncture is seen as part of the practice of 'Toyo Igaku', 'Oriental' or 'east Asian' medicine. While the term Toyo Igaku generally refers to all forms of traditional medicine in Japan, it recognizes the historical and modern tradition of the separate practice of acupuncture, moxibustion, massage and herbal medicines. In Japan, acupuncture, moxibustion and massage (anma, shiatsu) are separately licensed but routinely practised together, with great plurality in the explanatory models and techniques of practice (for discussions of the development of this plurality see Birch and Felt (1999) and Manaka (1994)). These are largely studied and practised independently from 'Kampo' or traditional herbal therapeutics. This separation is not only based on tradition but also nineteenth century legislation that requires practitioners of Kampo to be western-trained physicians or pharmacists, which most acupuncturists are not (Lock, 1980: 19). Thus acupuncture and moxibustion are mostly practised independently of traditional herbal medicine. In the west we also find terms such as 'Oriental medicine' or 'traditional east Asian medicine' used to refer to the broad array of traditional therapies that primarily originated in China. These terms are used in an effort to be inclusive of all traditions of practice from the 'Orient'.

Thus different terms are used in reference to the practice of acupuncture. These terms express different points of view, whereby acupuncture is for example:

1. An inseparable part of a larger medicine ('Chinese medicine', 'traditional Chinese medicine, TCM' or 'Oriental medicine'); where acupuncture is usually combined with herbal medicine, which is more popular in East Asia than acupuncture (Hillier and Jewell, 1983: 291; Sivin, 1987: 179; Unschuld, 1992: 55; Tsutani, 1993); *or*
2. A separate and distinct but related form of traditional medicine, for example 'meridian therapy' (Fukushima, 1991).

This has obvious consequences on how to understand acupuncture in the modern context. A range of opinions have developed where acupuncture is viewed as part of a whole system of medicine (e.g. see Liu, 1988b), an independently functioning system of medicine (e.g. see Shudo, 1990; Fukushima, 1991), or simply a set of techniques to be incorporated into biomedical practice (for western examples see Melzack, 1984; Baldry, 1989; Gaupp *et al.*, 1989; Chapman and Gunn, 1990; Ulett, 1992).

Historically acupuncture and moxibustion have been used in a variety of different ways to treat a large number of health problems. There has been a strong emphasis on applying treatment to correct the perceived physiological problems thought to cause the particular symptoms that a patient presents. Historically there have been many schools of thought regarding how and what are labelled as the physiological problems (for discussions of some of these variations, see Birch and Felt, 1999; Kaptchuk, 1985; Manaka *et al.*, 1995; MacPherson and Kaptchuk, 1997). In both the historical and modern literature there has also been an equally significant emphasis on applying treatment to relieve or correct specific symptoms, a fact that many modern practitioners have appeared to ignore, deny, or not understand (Coan *et al.*, 1980; Hansen and Hansen, 1983; Diebschlag, 1993). However, such claims are at odds with the historical facts. Many examples of 'symptomatic' acupuncture treatment exist, dating from the earliest texts to the present (e.g. see Birch, 1997). In the historical literature one finds a broad range of uses dating from the earliest important texts to more recent important historical texts, where acupuncture is used in what is called a 'formulary' or 'symptomatic' approach. It is thus not correct to label such approaches as 'non-traditional', to imply that they are not part of the traditional practice of acupuncture, or that they represent an inferior form of practice. Both approaches exist in East Asian acupuncture. For many acupuncturists in East Asia there is an idealized method of practice that does not focus primarily on relieving symptoms (e.g. see Liu, 1988b; Shudo, 1990; Fukushima, 1991; Manaka *et al.*, 1995), whereas for others acupuncture is used to relieve specific symptoms (e.g. see Hyodo, 1986; So, 1987; Serizawa and Kusumi, 1988). While there is polarization in the western literature around what appear to be two irreconcilable approaches to practice, this too is not in keeping with the historical literature. These two approaches were routinely used together like 'two wheels on an axle' (Manaka *et al.*, 1995: 156). In China this was called the 'zhibenfa' (root treatment) and 'zhibiaofa' (branch or symptomatic treatment), and in Japan, the 'honchiho' and 'hyochiho' respectively. Traditionally, the basic physiological models on which judgements are made about the 'zhibenfa' were rooted in the ancient Chinese theories of 'qi' and what Unschuld has called the 'Medicine of Systematic Correspondence' (Unschuld, 1985: 51ff). There are many descriptions of these various models, so rather than repeat them we will briefly discuss a number of key concepts that are central to the study of traditionally based acupuncture. Treatments based on these theories were complemented by empirically revised treatments to target the specific symptoms, which require little discussion.

Acupuncture is frequently described as a form of 'holistic' medicine quite different from western medicine (e.g. see Larre *et al.*, 1986: 19ff; Hammer, 1990; Beinfield and Korngold, 1991; Bensoussan, 1991: 2; Cassidy, 1995; World Health Organization, 1995). There are also claims that acupuncture has a long continuous almost unvarying history of use (e.g. see Veith, 1949: 70; Connelly, 1979: 5; Larre *et al.*, 1986: 19, 27 especially; Gaupp *et al.*, 1989: 182; NASCAOM, 1989; Carlsson and Sjolund, 1994; Yang and Liu, 1994: v). However, scholarly study of acupuncture in East Asia has found that the 'paradigm' of acupuncture is more complex than is frequently thought. It has both holistic and non-holistic components that co-exist side by side; further, its history is so long and complex that it becomes difficult to describe a single paradigm in acupuncture (Unschuld, 1987, 1992). The history of acupuncture evidences multiple traditions, often contradictory, with many ideas and methods, rather than continuous or coherent models of practice extending back two millenia (for descriptions of this history, see e.g. Epler, 1980; Lu and Needham, 1980; Hillier and Jewell, 1983; Unschuld, 1985, 1987, 1992; Wong and Wu, 1985; Sivin, 1987). Thus claims of a single continuous model of practice from historical times to the present, of acupuncture having a paradigm that is totally different from that of western medicine, or of acupuncture being purely holistic are not in keeping with established historical facts (Unschuld, 1985, 1987, 1992). The history and nature of acupuncture is more complex than this.

Traditional explanatory models and concepts

For all the diversity of approaches, underlying almost all forms of East Asian acupuncture is a set of shared preconceptions and premises. Essentially the traditional explanatory models underpinning acupuncture suggested that all things in the world are composed of qi (see discussions in Needham, 1956: 40–41; Porkert, 1974: 166ff; Unschuld, 1985: 67ff; Larre *et al.*, 1986: 49ff; Sivin, 1987: 46–47; Matsumoto and Birch, 1988: 83, 90–91; Klarer and Kaptchuk, 1997), where material objects including the human body are thought to be condensations of qi (see discussions in Needham, 1956: 76; Matsumoto and Birch, 1988: 114). Qi is constantly in flux, so that everything is always changing, which opens up the possibility of change. Qi is also what animates living things and consequently it is disturbances in qi that cause health problems (see discussions in Needham, 1956: 76; Unschuld, 1985: 67ff; Chiu, 1986: 84ff; Sivin, 1987: 48ff; Matsumoto and Birch, 1988: 84). Initially qi was seen as an undifferentiated whole, that, for the purposes of more detailed medical description, had to be categorized into multiple subsets (Chiu, 1986: 92ff). Thus qi as the basis of life was divided into a set of interrelated forms each with their different functions, movements and characteristics (Chiu, 1986: 85ff; Sivin, 1987: 149ff; see also Porkert, 1974: 168–176 for examples of the many forms of qi). The maintenance and production of these various forms of qi are brought about through the viscera and bowel organs, each of which have their own qi, and are responsible for other forms of qi (Table 1.1).

All mental and emotional states were related to qi, fostering a model

Table 1.1 Zang-fu organs

Zang (viscera)	*Fu (bowel)*
qi – production and storage	decompose food and convey waste
fei – lungs	da chang – large intestine
pi – spleen	wei – stomach
xin – heart	xiao chang – small intestine
gan – liver	dan – gallbladder
shen – kidneys	pang guang – bladder
xin bao luo – pericardium also known as 'xin zhu', the 'heart master' or 'heart governor'	san jiao – triple burner (see Wiseman and Ellis, 1985:91–92; Sivin, 1987: 124–126)

Table 1.2 Channel systems

Type	*Name*	*No.*	*Function*
jing mai	regular channels	12	circulate ying qi; each connected to 2 or more organs; each has their own acupoints
luo mai	connecting vessels	15	secondary channels for qi circulation (intersect regular channels)
jing bie	channel divergences	12	secondary channels for qi circulation (intersect regular channels)
jing jin	channel sinews	12	associated with body musculature
qi jing mai	extraordinary vessels	8	qi reservoirs, regulate qi distribution; 2 have own acupoints, 6 intersect regular channels

whereby there was not a sharp dichotomy between mind and body (Chiu, 1986). In this basic model, health and disease were not thought of as objective states, rather they reflect a dynamic state involving the tension and interaction of multiple components. The 'diagnosis' was made after collecting a variety of naked sense observations about the patient and synthesizing them into a pattern (see below). These 'diagnoses' were not reflective of some objective state or condition, such methods of classification had not developed. The diagnoses were generally predictors of treatment (see below), in so far as they led to treatment, and carried more the sense of prognosis than diagnosis.

Qi circulates in the body in regular patterns as 'ying qi' (construction or nourishing qi), through set pathways, the 'jing mai', in the system of 'jing luo' or channels and connecting vessels, with systems of secondary pathways and storage trajectories (e.g. the 'luo mai', 'jing jin', 'jing bie', 'qi jing ba mai'; Table 1.2).

There are 12 primary jing mai or channels, each associated with a specific zang or fu organ, and each with their own set of 'kong xue' or 'jing xue' acupuncture points, or more accurately acu-holes (Table 1.3).

The secondary (qi jing mai) pathways with their own acupoints are the ren mai – conception vessel (24 points) – and the du mai – governing

Table 1.3 The 12 channels and their major correspondencies

Arm/leg	*Yin–yang*	*Primary organ*	*Secondary organ*	*Number of acupoints*
arm	tai (greater) yin	lungs	large intestine	11
arm	yang ming (brightness)	large intestine	lungs	20
leg	yang ming	stomach	spleen	45
leg	tai yin	spleen	stomach	21
arm	shao (lesser) yin	heart	small intestine	9
arm	tai (greater) yang	small intestine	heart	19
leg	tai yang	bladder	kidneys	67
leg	shao yin	kidneys	bladder	27
arm	jue (absolute) yin	pericardium	san jiao	9
arm	shao (lesser) yang	san jiao	pericardium	23
leg	shao yang	gallbladder	liver	44
leg	jue yin	liver	gallbladder	14

vessel (28 points). Another form of qi, the 'wei qi' (defensive qi), was said to move across the body surface, helping protect the body from pathogenic influences, in particular environmental or climatic factors. Six major pathogenic influences were described, wind, cold, damp, heat, dryness and summerheat (Wiseman and Ellis, 1985: 96–101; Fukushima, 1991: 69–71). Exposure or overexposure to one or more of these influences can cause disruption of the circulating qi and eventually functional disruptions inside the body, gastrointestinal functions for example. These influences were known as 'xie qi' (literally 'evil qi'), referring to their disruptive effects upon the qi of the patient.

In the historical literature on acupuncture, additional factors were described as disrupting either the circulation of qi or various functional states of the qi systems. Of note are influences resulting from dietary, exercise and sexual habits. Overeating injures the spleen. Different flavoured foods when consumed inappropriately can disrupt organ functions, saltiness affects the kidneys, spiciness the lungs, sour the liver, sweet the spleen and bitter the heart. Also of note were influences resulting from the expression (or repression) of emotions, in particular anger, which affects the liver, fear which affects the kidneys, sadness the lungs, worrying the spleen and joy the heart. The aetiology of disease was often seen in relation to disruptions of the circulation of the qi, and/or the functions of each of the organs due to these various internal (e.g. emotional) or external (e.g. climatic) factors.

The systems of organs and channels were categorized according to whether they are 'yin' or 'yang' in nature. Yin–yang theory is simultaneously a cosmological theory for all things in nature, a theory describing the fundamental characteristics and interactions of all things in nature, a method of categorizing all things (Table 1.4), all of which lead to a series of regulatory descriptions of how parts within a whole interact and function.

For good discussions of the multiple descriptions of yin–yang theory, and for elaborations of yin–yang theories, see Needham (1956: 273ff), Porkert (1974: 9–43), Sivin (1987: 59ff), Unschuld (1985: 55–58) and Wiseman and Ellis (1985: 3–9). The 'zang' yin organs have the

Table 1.4 Yin–yang correspondencies

Yin	*Yang*
shaded side of mountain	sunny side of mountain
cool / cold	warm / hot
dark	light
heavy	light
passive	active
female	male
internal portions	external portions
insufficient	excessive
inferior half of the body	superior half of the body
anterior half of the body	posterior half of the body
zang organs	fu organs
yin channels: tai yin, shao yin, jue yin	yang channels: tai yang, shao yang, yang ming

characteristics of storage, primarily producing and storing qi; the 'fu' yang organs have the characteristics of movement-transportation, and primarily decompose food and convey waste (e.g. see Wiseman and Ellis, 1985: 65–93). The 12 primary jing mai are classified according to whether they are on the arm or leg and whether they are yin or yang, with subdivisions of each (Table 1.3). Everything has both yin and yang components, for example in 'zhong yi' there is extensive discussion of the yin and yang functions of each organ, such as 'kidney yin' and 'kidney yang' (e.g. see Wiseman and Ellis, 1985: 65–87). Many yin things are paired with yang things (e.g. the lung with the large intestine channels). These dual aspects and pairings are simultaneously syntagonistic and antagonistic, whereby the correlated yin and yang try to counterbalance each other, helping to maintain a 'balanced' state, and can produce change in the other, much like the two ends of a see-saw, one goes up, the other down.

The jing mai and zang fu are further described in relation to the 'wu xing' or five-phase (sometimes known as five element) theory, which, like yin–yang, is simultaneously a cosmological theory, a system for classifying all things, a system for describing fundamental characteristics and interactions of all things and a description of regulatory interactions within whole systems (for discussions of these multiple descriptions, and elaborations of five-phase theory see Needham, 1956: 232ff, especially 253–265; Porkert, 1974: 43–54; Unschuld, 1985: 58–61; Wiseman and Ellis, 1985: 10–18; Sivin, 1987: 70ff; Birch and Friedman, 1989). The relationships of each phase to the other, and hence things that correlate within one phase to things within another phase, are much more complex than yin–yang pairings and interactions. Each phase is interacting with the other four at all times in four different patterns:

1. The engendering cycle, whereby each phase reinforces the next in the engendering sequence: wood→fire→earth→metal→water→wood. If wood increases this tends to cause an increase in fire (wood engenders fire).
2. The restraining cycle, whereby each phase restrains another in set patterns: wood restrains earth; earth restrains water; water restrains fire; fire restrains metal; metal restrains wood. If wood increases this tends to produce a decrease in earth (wood restrains earth), and if wood decreases this tends to produce an increase in earth.
3. The counter-engendering cycle: wood→water→metal→earth→fire→wood.
4. The counter-restraining cycle: wood→metal→fire→water→earth→wood.

Table 1.5 lists some of the major five-phase correspondences.

Within each phase, each corresponding thing is related to all other corresponding things within the phase. A change in one can potentially create changes in other corresponding things in the phase.

The circulation of qi in the systems of channels affects organ functions; the functions of the organs affect the circulation of qi in the channels. Yin–yang and five-phase theories describe fundamental interactions and regulatory functions within the whole system. When particular organs

Table 1.5 Five-phase correspondencies

	Wood	*Fire*	*Earth*	*Metal*	*Water*
zang organs + channels	liver	heart/pericardium	spleen	lungs	kidneys
fu organs + channels	gallbladder	small intestine/ triple burner	stomach	large intestine	bladder
colours	blue/green	red	yellow	white	blue/black
tastes	sour	bitter	sweet	spicy	salty
odours	greasy/oily	scorched	sweet	raw flesh	rancid
tones	shouting	laughing	singing	weeping	groaning
sense organs	eyes	tongue	mouth	nose	ears
tissues	sinews	vessels	flesh	body hair	bones
disposition	anger	joy	preoccupation	sorrow	fear
climate	wind	heat	damp	dry	cold

lose their normal functions, they most commonly become 'xu', vacuous, or 'shi', replete. The qi circulating in the channels can be vacuous, replete or 'zhi', 'stagnant'. Treatments in these traditional models are aimed at supplementing 'bu', what is vacuous; draining 'xie', what is replete; or rectifying and moving 'li', what is stagnant (for elaborations of treatment principles see Wiseman and Ellis, 1985: 371–450; Shudo, 1990: 190–198; Fukushima, 1991: 157–166; Manaka *et al.*, 1995). The 'zhiben fa' (root treatment) aims primarily at correcting observed problems in 'qi function' (at the level of the zang-fu) or 'qi circulation' (at the level of the jing-luo). The acupuncture treatments target specific acupoints/acu-holes that have been described as effecting the needed changes in qi function or qi circulation, utilizing appropriate techniques to achieve those goals.

The above is a greatly simplified overview of how the whole much more complex set of traditionally modelled systems work, it captures the basic aspects involved in most traditionally based models of practice. Additionally, there are also models of practice whereby acupuncture points are treated based primarily on empirical uses, often informed by historical empirical descriptions (e.g. see So, 1985; Serizawa and Kusumi, 1988; Debata, 1990).

The diversity of current models and methods of practice

A brief review of texts from various East Asian countries quickly reveals the diversity of explanatory models, models of practice and techniques used by acupuncturists (e.g. O'Connor and Bensky, 1981; Cheng, 1987; Fukushima, 1991; Manaka *et al.*, 1995). Recent publications in the east have further elaborated this diversity (e.g. see Birch, 1998; Macpherson and Kaptchuk, 1997). There is considerable diversity both within and between various East Asian countries in the practice of acupuncture. Tables 1.6 and 1.7 tabulate examples of the multiplicity of treatment models found in practice. Table 1.6 presents examples from the historical and modern literature of the basic approaches to treatment, traditionally called 'zhiben fa' and 'zhibiao fa'.

Table 1.6 Examples of zhi ben/zhi biao treatment approaches

	Historical examples	*Modern examples*
zhi ben root treatments	*Huang Di Nei Jing Su Wen* (circa 200) – see Liao, 1992 Huang-fu Mi (282) – see Yang and Chace, 1994	Fukushima, 1991 Shudo, 1990 Wiseman and Ellis, 1985
zhi biao symptom control treatments	*Huang Di Nei Jing Su Wen* (circa 200) – see Liao, 1992 Huang-fu Mi (282) – see Yang and Chace, 1994	Serizawa and Kusumi, 1988 So, 1987 Ulett, 1992
zhi ben and zhi biao treatments	Huang-fu Mi (282) – see Yang and Chace, 1994 Yang Ji-zhou (1601) see Yang and Liu, 1994	Manaka *et al.*, 1995 Soulie de Morant, 1994

Notice how the same historical source (Chapter 41 of the *Su Wen*) describes separate zhiben and zhibiao approaches to the treatment of low back pain (Liao, 1992).

Table 1.7 presents examples of the diverse explanatory models found in the modern international practice of acupuncture.

The grouping of models is only approximate as some might argue that some models, such as that of 'zhong yi' acupuncture, may be more accurately classified under 'mixture of traditional and modern explanations'.

While Tables 1.6 and 1.7 clearly do not cover all models of practice in the field of acupuncture, they at least give a clear picture of the diversity of treatment strategies (general/root treatment focused, symptom relief focused or both), and explanatory models (traditional, scientific, a combination or other). Clearly this is a heterogeneous field of enormous complexity.

Patient assessment in historically based models of practice

We have seen that there are many ideas about the nature of acupuncture. While the traditional forms of acupuncture are usually anchored in

Table 1.7 Examples of varied explanatory models of acupuncture

traditional explanations only	Anon, 1980; Wiseman and Ellis, 1985; Cheng, 1987; Liu, 1988a; Shudo, 1990; Fukushima, 1991
mixture of traditional and modern explanations	Mann, 1974; Nakatani and Yamashita, 1977; O'Connor and Bensky, 1981; Liao *et al.*, 1994; Helms, 1995; Manaka *et al.*, 1995
modern anatomically based explanations only	Baldry, 1989; Debata, 1990; Ulett, 1992; Seem, 1993
unique ideas	Zhang, 1979; Nogier, 1983; Suehara, 1985

traditional explanatory models that revolve around the concepts of qi, yin–yang, wu xing, zang-fu, jing-luo, etc., it has also been shown that there have been many interpretations of, and models based on, these concepts. This section will examine the diagnostic methods that have been historically used to assess patients, and which guide treatment decisions.

Acupuncture originally developed in a virtually technology-free culture, thus this traditional medicine depended on naked sense observations to gather data about patient problems. Certain philosophical views of the world present at that time guided how health, disease and treatment were viewed and conceived. Since its inception, the historical texts describing its use have guided its practice into the modern period. Thus the history of acupuncture also manifests an evolution of these early data-gathering methods and of the interpretive context of the data gathered about each patient. As we have seen above, there are now many models of practice that utilize these methods in variant ways (for examples of this variety see Kaptchuk, 1983; Shudo, 1990; Manaka *et al.*, 1995).

As human beings we have five primary senses, each of which can be used to gather data about the world and thus patients – the visual, auditory, olfactory, gustatory and tactile senses. Through the centuries, different historical texts placed differing degrees of emphasis on each of these senses, but basically recommended following a systematic data-gathering method, the so-called four inspections. Patient data are gathered through:

(i) visual inspection;
(ii) listening/smelling;
(iii) questioning; and
(iv) palpation.

Relevant data are collected and analysed within the theoretical frameworks used by the practitioner, according to descriptions of the zang-fu organs, the channels, five phases, yin–yang, etc. Using the four inspections, data are gathered relative to the functions and observed pathology of each organ, the pathways and observed pathology of each channel, the organ/channel, five-phase and yin–yang correspondencies. Thus, for example, under visual inspection one attempts to classify the colour of the patient according to the five-phase colours (Table 1.5). One might also examine the shape, size, colour of the tongue body, and the colour and texture of the coating on the tongue within the yin–yang framework of the traditional Chinese medical acupuncture model (e.g. see Chen and Chen, 1989). Under listening/smelling one attempts to classify the tones of voice and body odour according to the five–phase correspondencies (Table 1.5). Under questioning, in addition to taking a medical history and family medical history, one asks additional questions in an attempt to identify problems that appear associated with one or more channels, organs, or match according to other five-phase correspondencies, such as preferences for one of the five tastes (Tables 1.4, 1.5 and 1.8).

Under palpation, in addition to palpation of acupoints, the channels

Table 1.8 Symptomatology of liver patterns in Chinese and Japanese traditional diagnoses

Ascendant activity if liver yang	*Liver vacuity*
rashness	liver disease
impatience	heaviness of the head
anger	eye problems
headache	lower back pain
dizziness	pain in the hip or knee joints
ocular rubor	pain along the medial aspect of the leg
dry mouth	urogenital disorders
insomnia	
palpitations	
pain in the lumbar region	
limp legs	

and a more systematic palpation of the abdomen (e.g. see Matsumoto and Birch, 1988), palpation of the radial arteries has been strongly emphasized and is a characteristic of most traditionally based models of practice. The radial arteries are palpated close to the wrists, three consecutive portions of each artery being palpated: at the radial notch and either side of it. The relative strengths of each position may be discriminated, as might the 'quality' of the pulses. A number of schools of practice today still use these pulse diagnosis methods. Since at least the first century, this method has been systematically described, with the findings classified according to problems of the organs, channels, qi, etc. Six positional diagnosis is prevalent in some models of practice (e.g. see Shudo, 1990; Fukushima, 1991), while discrimination of up to 28 different pulse qualities are more prevalent in other models of practice (e.g. see Kaptchuk, 1983; Wiseman and Ellis, 1985; Ikeda and Ikeda, 1991).

The practitioner collects observations and information for each patient which come from a broad spectrum of areas of that patient's life. These are then classified or organized to arrive at a 'pattern' of diagnosis (in Chinese 'zheng', Japanese 'akashi' or 'sho') which is capable of explaining a wide range of symptoms and events of concern to the patient. While this diagnostic process and the traditional diagnosis have similarities to biomedicine (Unschuld, 1987, 1992), they also contain components that are quite different in nature from a western biomedical diagnosis. The biomedical diagnosis attempts to arrive at an objective scientific description or label of disease, which in turn opens up to selection of an appropriate treatment, if one exists. The traditionally based acupuncture diagnosis makes no effort to objectively describe disease, rather it seeks to classify various signs and symptoms according to traditional notions of health and disease, such as qi, yin–yang, jing-luo, etc. (e.g. see Wiseman and Ellis, 1985; Shudo, 1990; Manaka *et al.*, 1995), eventually categorizing these as some kind of pattern or conformation, which in turn **always** has a prescribed treatment associated with it. The guaranteed matching of treatment to diagnosis has led some to speculate that, at the very least, we can conclude that the traditionally based acupuncture diagnostic assessment focuses on determining what treatment should be administered (Friedman *et al.*, 1997; Tsutani and

Birch, in preparation). Despite recent Chinese investigations (e.g. see Chen, 1988; Xie, 1988), there is still inadequate data one way or the other to allow for a determination of the actual nature of these diagnostic assessments. It is reasonable to propose that the traditionally based diagnosis may be a heuristic device for selecting treatment, or a stepping stone in the therapeutic process, but does not necessarily describe an objective entity as biomedicine attempts to do.

Many different symptoms and patient complaints may correspond within each traditionally based pattern of diagnosis. Table 1.8 lists 11 major symptoms associated with the Chinese zhong yi 'zheng' of 'ascendant activity of liver yang' (Wiseman and Ellis, 1985: 259) and seven major symptoms associated with the Japanese 'sho' 'liver vacuity' (Shudo, 1990: 133). Similarly, a group of patients with the same western medical diagnosis, for example, tension headache, can manifest one of a number of different patterns commonly associated with the problem of tension headache. Table 1.9 lists the ten types of headache that can be found in a recent textbook of traditional Chinese medicine (Wu and Fischer, 1997: 162–173).

Therapeutic techniques and methods

The choice of therapeutic interventions and the differences in how needles and moxa are used also manifest a wide range of variations. Historically, the *Huang Di Nei Jing Ling Shu* described nine kinds of needles, each of which was used for different purposes, two of which were not inserted, instead being pressed or rubbed on the skin (for descriptions of the nine needles see Birch and Ida (1998). The oldest needles were said to be of stone (the 'bian') (Lu and Needham, 1980: 69ff), but fell out of use once metal needles became available. The oldest metal needles appear to have been made of bronze, silver and gold (Lu and Needham, 1980: 69ff), though now stainless steel needles are used by the vast majority of acupuncturists. Of the nine needles described in the *Ling Shu*, the filiform needle is by far the most commonly used; most of the other eight needles only find common use within certain traditionally based schools of practice. Many gauges and lengths of filiform needle can be found, commonly ranging from gauge 0.12 mm to 0.30 mm, but the needles can be wider gauge. The depth of insertion also varies, from routine very shallow needling (1–2 mm) to routine deeper needling, depending upon the points needled (5–60 mm). Once inserted many different techniques of manipulation can be used, giving quite different subjective sensations for the patient. Additional electrical stimulation of

Table 1.9 Ten traditional Chinese medicine categories of headache

wind – cold headache	wind – heat headache
wind – dampness headache	liver yang headache
kidney yin vacuity headache	kidney yang vacuity headache
qi vacuity headache	blood vacuity headache
phlegm – turbidity headache	blood stasis headache

the needles is also commonly used. Filiform needles are also used by some practitioners without actual penetration of the skin, where the needle tip is held at or just above the skin surface to produce benefit. Various other kinds of needles have been developed, including the 'plum blossom needle', the 'press-tack needle' and the 'intradermal needle'.

Table 1.10 gives examples of the various needle types and methods that can be found in modern practice.

More than 50 different moxibustion methods have also been described in the historical literature (Zhang and Geng, 1991: 10), with a variety of common methods surviving into modern practice. Moxa may be used by burning it directly on the skin (direct moxa), which can be used to blister or not blister the point, it may be applied on top of a variety of substances placed on the skin, such as ginger, garlic, soybean paste, or it may be applied indirectly over the skin, where it is rolled up into a roll and held above the skin surface. It is also applied on top of the handle of the acupuncture needle to produce additive effects to the needling (e.g. see

Table 1.10 Examples of the diverse methods employed in acupuncture

needling with 'de qi' type stimulation – sensations of 'soreness, numbness, heaviness, distention' (Cheng, 1987: 326) or 'sharp, pulling, electric, tingling, heavy, pulsing, spreading, pricking, aching or hot' (Vincent *et al.*,1989)	Anon, 1980; Bensky, 1981; Cheng, 1987; O'Connor and So, 1987; Soulie de Morant, 1994
needling with no de qi type stimulation	Zhang, 1979; Akabane, 1986; Shudo, 1990; Fukushima, 1991; Manaka *et al.*,1995
shallow needling	Shudo, 1990; Fukushima, 1991; Birch and Ida, 1998
non-inserted needling	Mori and Yoneyama, 1983; Fukushima, 1991; Birch and Ida, 1998
needling to stimulate nerve structures	O'Connor and Bensky, 1981: 467–469; Serizawa and Kusumi, 1988; Baldry, 1989; Ulett, 1992
electroacupuncture	O'Connor and Bensky, 1981; Shimizu, 1986; Cheng, 1987; Baldry, 1989; Ulett, 1992; Helms, 1995
tiny electrical stimulation	Matsumoto and Birch, 1988; Manaka *et al.*, 1995
two-metal contact or magnets	Nagatomo, 1976; Chen, 1979
moxibustion	Anon, 1980; O'Connor and Bensky, 1981; Irie, 1980; Cheng, 1987; So, 1987; Ellis *et al.*, 1988; Manaka *et al.*, 1995; Birch and Ida, 1998
cupping	O'Connor and Bensky, 1981; Wang and Ren, 1985; Cheng, 1987; Meguro, 1991; Birch and Ida, 1998
scarification by gua sha	So, 1987; Nielsen, 1995
bloodletting	Maruyama and Kudo, 1982; Wang and Ren, 1985; Birch and Ida, 1998
surgical applications	O'Connor and Bensky, 1981

Irie, 1980; O'Connor and Bensky, 1981; Manaka *et al.*, 1995; Birch and Ida, 1998). Other additional treatment methods may be used, such as suction pressure or 'cupping', and scarification by 'gua sha'. Table 1.10 presents examples of the techniques used in modern international acupuncture practice.

Were the same patient to present to practitioners of different schools or models of acupuncture practice, it is clear that the patient would receive quite different treatments from the practitioners of each (e.g. see Birch, 1997). There would be variety in the descriptive labels given by each system, and an even greater variety of treatment techniques. Needling for example is very different. Subjective sensations in the patient upon needling are prescribed in one system (e.g. Cheng, 1987; Ellis *et al.*, 1988) and yet prohibited in another (e.g. Shudo, 1990; Fukushima, 1991). Needling depths range from 0.75 to 3.75 cm in one system to 0.1 to 0.4 cm in another (Birch, 1997). In general, treatment involves the insertion of a number of needles, often with the addition of the various techniques, combined to rectify the pattern and/or to relieve the symptoms. Each treatment combination is couched within the model of practice used and varies according to individual patient differences.

Conclusion

This chapter shows that while there are common threads that run through traditionally based systems of acupuncture, there is also a great deal of heterogeneity. Acupuncture has been a diverse tradition with many voices and styles both in the historical and modern periods. As this type of health care becomes more easily available in the industrial western world, it is important that the romantic view of the unified coherent 'all knowing' east does not come to obscure the richness and complexity of this tradition. While a critical examination may seem daunting, it is the only option available if we are to encounter the potential depth of acupuncture's contribution to a new cosmopolitan medicine.

References

Akabane, K. (1986). *Hinaishin Ho (Intradermal Needle Method)*, 12th edn. Yokosuka: Ido no Nippon Company.

Anon (1980). *Essentials of Chinese Acupuncture*. Beijing: Foreign Languages Press.

Baldry, P. E. (1989). *Acupuncture, Trigger Points and Musculoskeletal Pain*. Edinburgh: Churchill Livingstone.

Beinfield, H. and Korngold, E. (1991). *Between Heaven and Earth*. New York: Ballantine Books.

Bensoussan, A. (1991). *The Vital Meridian*. Edinburgh: Churchill Livingstone.

Birch, S. (1997). An Exploration with Proposed Solutions of the Problems and Issues in Conducting Clinical Research in Acupuncture. PhD thesis, University of Exeter.

Birch, S. (1998). Diversity and acupuncture: acupuncture is not a coherent or historically stable tradition.. In *Examining Complementary Medicine: the Sceptical Holist* (A. J. Vickers, ed.). Cheltenham: Stanley Thomas, 45–63.

Birch, S. and Felt, R. (1999). *Understanding Acupuncture*. Edinburgh: Churchill Livingstone.

Birch, S. and Friedman, M. (1989). On the development of a mathematical model for the 'laws' of the five phases. *Am. J. Acupunct.*, **17,** 361–366.

Birch, S. and Ida, J. (1998). *Japanese Acupuncture: A Clinical Guide.* Brookline, Massachusetts: Paradigm Publications.

Birch, S. and Tsutani, K. (1996). A bibliometrical study of English-language materials on acupuncture. *Comp. Ther. Med.*, **4,** 172–177.

Carlsson, C. P. O. and Sjolund, B. H. (1994). Acupuncture and subtypes of chronic pain: assessment of long-term results. *Clin. J. Pain*, **10,** 290–295.

Cassidy, C. (1995). Social science theory and methods in the study of alternative and complementary medicine. *J. Alt. Comp. Med.*, **1,** 19–40.

Chapman, C. R. and Gunn, C. C. (1990). Acupuncture. In *The Management of Pain*, vol. I, 2nd edn. (J. J. Bonica, ed.) pp. 1805–1821. Philadelphia: Lea and Febiger.

Chen, Z. (1979). *Ci Liao Fa (Magnet Treatment Methods)*. Hunan: Science and Technology.

Chen, Z. L. (1988). Development of research on tongue diagnosis. *Chin. J. Integrated Med.*, **8**(special issue 2), 104–108.

Chen, Z. L. and Chen, M. F. (1989). *The Essence and Scientific Background of Tongue Diagnosis.* Long Beach: Oriental Healing Arts Institute.

Cheng, X. N. (1987). *Chinese Acupuncture and Moxibustion*. Beijing: Foreign Languages Press.

Chiu, M. L. (1986). Mind, Body, and Illness in a Chinese Medical Tradition. PhD thesis, Harvard University.

Coan, R., Wong, G., Ku, S. L. *et al.* (1980). The acupuncture treatment of low back pain: a randomized controlled treatment. *Am. J. Chin. Med.*, **VIII,** 181–189.

Connelly, D. (1979). *Traditional Acupuncture: The Law of the Five Elements.* Colombia, Maryland: The Centre for Traditional Acupuncture.

Debata, A. (1990). *Kaigyo Shinkyushi no tameno Shinsatsuho to Chiryo (Diagnosis and Treatment of Sciatica for the Private Practitioner Acupuncturist)*, 4th edn. Yokosuka: Ido no Nippon Sha.

Diebschlag, F. (1993). Placebo acupuncture. *Eur. J. Oriental Med.*, **1**(2), 12–17.

Ellis, A., Wiseman, N. and Boss, K. (1988). *Fundamentals of Chinese Acupuncture.* Brookline, Massachusetts: Paradigm Publications.

Epler, D. C. (1980). Bloodletting in early Chinese medicine and its relation to the origin of acupuncture. *Bull. History Med.*, **54,** 337–367.

Ergil, M. C. (1993). Letter to the editor. *J. Acupuncture Soc. N. Y.*, **1**(2–3), 23–26.

Ergil, M. C. (1994). Medical education in China. *CCAOM News*, **1**(1), 3–5.

Friedman, M., Birch, S. and Tiller, W. A. (1997). Mathematical modelling as a tool in basic research in acupuncture. *J. Alt. Comp. Med.*, **3**(suppl 1), S89–S99.

Fukushima, K. (1991). *Meridian Therapy*. Tokyo: Toyo Hari Medical Association.

Gaupp, L. A., Flinn, D. E. and Weddige, R. L. (1989). Adjunctive treatment techniques. In *Handbook of Chronic Pain Management* (C. D. Tollison, ed.) pp. 174–196. Baltimore: Williams and Wilkins.

Hammer, L. (1990). *Dragon Rises, Red Bird Flies*. New York: Station Hill Press.

Hansen, P. E. and Hansen, J.H. (1983). Acupuncture treatment of chronic facial pain – a controlled cross-over trial. *Headache*, **23,** 66–69.

Helms, J. (1995). *Acupuncture Energetics: A Clinical Approach for Physicians*. Berkley: Medical Acupuncture Publishers.

Hillier, S. M. and Jewell, J. A. (1983) *Health Care and Traditional Chinese Medicine in China 1800–1982*. London: Routledge and Kegan Paul.

Hyodo, M. (1986). Acupuncture therapeutic points suited to diseases and disorders. *Nihon Ryodoraku Jiritsushinkei Gakkai Zasshi*, **31,** 4–5.

Ikeda, T. and Ikeda, M. (1991). *Zo Fu Keiraku Karamita Yakuho to Shinkyu*, vol. 5. Imahari City: Kampo In Yo Kai.

Irie, S. (1980). *Fukaya Kyu Ho. Fukaya's Moxa Method.* Tokyo: Shizensha.

Ishihara, T. (1983). A compilation of pre-Meiji-era acupuncture related classical literature. *Keiraku Chiryo*, **72,** 8–45.

Kaptchuk, T. J. (1983). *The Web That Has No Weaver.* New York: Congdon and Weed.

Kaptchuk, T. J. (1985). Introduction. In *Fundamentals of Chinese Medicine* (N. Wiseman and A. Ellis, eds). Brookline, Massachusetts: Paradigm Publications.

Klarer, S. and Kaptchuk, T. J. (1997). Qi. In *Encyclopedia of the History of Science, Technology, and Medicine in Non-West Cultures* (H. Selin ed.), pp. 832–833. Dordrecht: Kluwer Academic Publishers.

Larre, C., Schatz, J. and Rochat de la Vallee, E. (1986). *Survey of Traditional Chinese Medicine.* Paris: l'Institute Ricci.

Liao, S. J. (1992). Acupuncture for low back pain. *Huang Di Nei Jing Su Wen. (Acupuncture and Electro-therapeutics Research International Journal)* **17,** 249–258.

Liao, S. J., Lee, M. H. M. and Ng, L. K. (1994). *Principles and Practice of Contemporary Acupuncture.* New York: Marcel Dekker.

Liu, B. Q. (1988). *Optimum Time for Acupuncture.* Jinan: Shandong Science and Technology Press.

Liu, Y. C. (1988). *The Essential Book of Traditional Chinese Medicine.* New York: Columbia University Press.

Lock, M. M. (1980). *East Asian Medicine in Urban Japan.* Berkley: University of California Press.

Lu, G. D. and Needham, J. (1980). *Celestial Lancets.* Cambridge: Cambridge University Press.

Maciocia, G. (1989). *Foundations of Chinese Medicine.* Edinburgh: Churchill Livingstone.

Macpherson, H. and Kaptchuk, T. J. (1997) *Acupuncture in Practice.* Edinburgh: Churchill Livingstone.

Manaka, Y. (1994). Japanese and Chinese acupuncture: similarities and differences. *North Am. J. Oriental Med.*, **1**(2), 5–9.

Manaka, Y., Itaya, K. and Birch, S. (1995). *Chasing the Dragon's Tail.* Brookline, Massachusetts: Paradigm Publications.

Mann, F. (1974). *Treatment of Disease by Acupuncture.* London: William Heinemann Medical Books.

Maruyama, M. and Kudo, K. (1982). *Shinpan Shiraku Ryoho.* Tokyo: Seki Bundo Publishing Company.

Matsumoto, K. and Birch, S. (1988). *Hara Diagnosis: Reflections on the Sea.* Brookline, Massachusetts: Paradigm Publications.

Meguro, A. (1991). *Kyukaku Ryoho,* 5th edn. Tokyo: Midori Shobo Publishing Company.

Melzack, R. (1984). Acupuncture and related forms of folk medicine. In *Textbook of Pain* (R. Melzack and P. D. Wall, eds), pp. 691–700. Edinburgh: Churchill Livingstone.

Mitchell, B. (1996). Educational and licensing requirements for acupuncturists. *J. Alt. Comp. Med.*, **2,** 33–35.

Mori, H. and Yoneyama, H. (1983). *Shoni Shin. Pediatric Acupuncture.* Yokosuka: Ido No Nippon Publishing Company.

Nagatomo, T. (1976). *Nagatomo MP Shinkyu Kuowa Hachiju Hachisyu. Mr. Nagatomo's 88 Lectures on Minus-plus Needle Therapy.* Kyoto: Shinkyu Shinkuokai Sha.

Nakagawa, Y. (1987). The present situation for acupuncture and moxibustion clinics and practitioners in Japan. *Ido no Nippon Mag.*, **46**(7), 102–107; **46**(8), 91–95.

Nakatani, Y. and Yamashita, K. (1977). *Ryodoraku Acupuncture.* Tokyo: Ryodoraku Research Institute.

NASCAOM, National Accreditation Commission for Schools and Colleges of Acupuncture and Oriental Medicine (1989). American acupuncture: a historical perspective. *J. Trad. Acupunct.* Spring 1989, 12–19.

Needham, J. (1956). *Science and Civilisation in China,* vol. II. Cambridge: Cambridge University Press.

Needham, J. and Lu, G. D. (1975). Problems of translation and modernisation of ancient Chinese technical terms. *Ann. Sci.*, **32,** 491–502.

Nielsen, A. (1995). *Gua Sha.* Edinburgh: Churchill Livingstone.

Nogier, P. F. M. (1983). *From Auriculotherapy to Auriculomedicine.* Saint-Ruffine: Maisonneuve.

O'Connor, J. and Bensky, D. (1981). *Acupuncture a Comprehensive Text.* Seattle: Eastland Press.

Porkert, M. (1974). *The Theoretical Foundations of Chinese Medicine.* Cambridge: MIT Press.

Rosenthal, M. M. (1987). *Health Care in the People's Republic of China: Moving Toward Modernization.* Boulder: Westview Press.

Seem, M. (1993). *A New American Acupuncture.* Boulder: Blue Poppy Press.

Serizawa, K. and Kusumi, M. (1988). *Clinical Acupuncture.* Tokyo: Japan Publications Inc.

Shimizu, K. (1986). Pressure pain points, diagnosis and treatments. *Ido no Nippon Mag.*, **45** (4), 315–324.

Shudo, D. (1990). *Japanese Classical Acupuncture: Introduction to Meridian Therapy.* Seattle: Eastland Press.

Sivin, N. (1987). *Traditional Medicine in Contemporary China.* Ann Arbor: Center for Chinese Studies, University of Michigan.

So, J. T. Y. (1985). *Book of Acupuncture Points.* Brookline, Massachusetts: Paradigm Publications.

So, J. T. Y. (1987). *Treatment of Disease with Acupuncture.* Brookline, Massachusetts: Paradigm Publications.

Sonoda, K. (1988). *Health and Illness in Changing Japanese Society.* Tokyo: University of Tokyo Press.

Soulie de Morant, G. (1994). *Chinese Acupuncture.* Brookline, Massachusetts: Paradigm Publications.

Suehara, I. (1985). *Genso Keiraku Ho; Fundamental Meridian Therapy.* Published privately by his Onso Shindangaku Kenkyujo Research Institute.

Tsutani, K. (1993). The evaluation of herbal medicines: an East Asian perspective. In *Clinical Research Methodology for Complementary Therapies* (G. T. Lewith and D. Aldridge, eds). London: Hodder and Stoughton.

Tsutani, K. and Birch, S. (in preparation). Evaluating complementary and alternative diagnostics.

Ulett, G. (1992). *Beyond Yin and Yang.* St Louis, Missouri: Warren H. Green Inc.

Unschuld, P. U. (1985). *Medicine in China: A History of Ideas.* Berkley: University of California Press.

Unschuld, P. U. (1986). *Medicine in China: Nan Ching the Classic of Difficult Issues.* Berkley: University of California Press.

Unschuld, P. U. (1987). Traditional Chinese medicine; some historical and epistemological reflections. *Soc. Sci. Med.*, **24,** 1023–1029.

Unschuld, P. U. (ed.) (1989). *Approaches to Traditional Chinese Medical Literature.* Dordrecht: Kluwer Academic Publishers.

Unschuld, P. U. (1990). *Forgotten Traditions of Ancient Chinese Medicine.* Brookline, Massachusetts: Paradigm Publications.

Unschuld, P. U. (1992). Epistemological issues and changing legitimation: traditional Chinese medicine in the twentieth century. In *Paths to Asian Medical Knowledge* (C. Leslie and A. Young, eds). Berkley: University of California Press.

Veith, I. (1949). *The Yellow Emperor's Classic of Internal Medicine.* Berkley: University of California Press.

Vincent, C. A., Richardson, P. H., Black, J. J. and Pither, C. E. (1989). The significance of needle placement site in acupuncture. *J. Psychosom. Res.*, **33,** 489–496.

Wang, F. Y. and Ren, H. Z. (1985) *Kyugyoku Ryoho, Cupping Therapy* (translated by Kaname Asakawa;) Ichikawa City: Toyo Gakujutsu Publishing Company.

World Health Organization (1985). *The Role of Traditional Medicine in Primary Health Care.* WPR/RC36/Technical_Discussions. Geneva: WHO.

World Health Organization (1995). *Guidelines for Clinical Research on Acupuncture.* Manila, Philippines: WHO.

Wiseman, N. (1995). *English–Chinese, Chinese–English Dictionary of Chinese Medicine.* Hunan: Hunan Science and Technology Publishers.

Wiseman, N. and Boss, K. (1990). *Glossary of Chinese Medical Terms and Acupuncture Points.* Brookline, Massachusetts: Paradigm Publications.

Wiseman, N. and Ellis, A. (1985). *Fundamentals of Chinese Medicine.* Brookline, Massachusetts: Paradigm Publications.

Wong, K. C. and Wu, L. T. (1985). *History of Chinese Medicine,* 2nd edn. Taipei: Southern Medical Materials.

Wu, Y. and Fischer, W. (1997). *Practical Therapeutics of Traditional Chinese Medicine.* Brookline, Massachusetts: Paradigm Publications.

Xie, Z. F. (1988). Researches on 'cold' and 'heat' in traditional Chinese medicine. *Chin. J. Integrated Med.,* **8**(special issue 2), 93–96.

Xue, Q. L. (chief editor) (1991). *The International Chinese Medicine Union Book Catalogue.* Beijing: Chinese Medical Ancient Books Publishing Company.

Yanagiya, S. (1948). *Shinkyu Ijutsu no Mon; An Introduction to the Medical Arts of Acupuncture and Moxibustion.* Yokosuka: Ido no Nippon sha.

Yang, S. Z. and Chace, C. (1994). *The Systematic Classic of Acupuncture and Moxibustion.* Boulder: Blue Poppy Press.

Yang, S. Z. and Liu, F. T. (1994). *The Divinely Responding Classic.* Boulder: Blue Poppy Press.

Zhang, F. R. and Geng, J. Y. (1991). *Zhong Guo Jiu Liao Xue.* Taipei: Zhi Yin Publishing Company.

Zhang, X. S. (1979). *Wan Ke Zhen; Wrist Ankle Acupuncture* (translated by Matsutane Sugi). Yokosuka: Ido no Nippon sha.

2

Western medical acupuncture

Jacqueline Filshie and Michael Cummings

Introduction and historical perspective

'Western acupuncture' is a term with a variety of potential meanings. The most literal interpretation invokes thoughts of geographical boundaries, but the term was probably introduced to distinguish a developing system of needle therapy from its traditional philosophical roots which happened to be in the east.

The authors of this text prefer to interpret 'western medical acupuncture' as the scientific application of acupuncture as a therapy following orthodox clinical diagnosis, whereas 'traditional Chinese acupuncture' (TCA) is an integral part of 'traditional Chinese medicine' (TCM) and therefore encompasses the multiple and often conflicting processes of diagnosis and treatment (see Chapter 1). It is important to note that the scientific evaluation of acupuncture is not restricted to the west (Han, 1987) and therefore adherence to a geographical definition is inappropriate. Probably a more accurate description of western medical acupuncture is a modern scientific approach to therapy involving dry needling of tissues, which has developed from the introduction and evaluation of TCA in the west.

Perhaps the most critical changes in the development of western acupuncture resulted from the application of scientific method. Science (Latin *scientia*, from *scire*, 'to know'), in its broadest meaning is the term used to denote systematized knowledge in any field, but applied usually to the organization of objectively verifiable sense experience (Boyer, 1994). In addition to the use of sophisticated language, the modification of behaviour based on reason as opposed to instinct is the key factor that distinguishes man from most other animals. Essentially it is the application of science that has led to the position of dominance of man over the rest of the species.

Modern scientific method was established by Galileo in the seventeenth century when he introduced systematic verification through planned experiments to the existing ancient methods of reasoning and deduction. This system was adopted by the scientific community throughout the globe, and with only the addition of statistical analysis it remains established practice today. Medical progress requires the constant reassessment and updating of a factual knowledge base. New hypotheses developed from clinical observation or reasoning are tested in order to enhance or refute that existing knowledge. The ethical practice of medicine requires the practitioner to understand and use scientific method.

A western view of the history and philosophy of acupuncture

Fossil evidence of trepanning indicates that man has used physical therapies in the treatment of disease since Neolithic times (circa 10 000 to 3500 BC). Acupuncture-like therapies have developed independently in different civilizations around the world. Children learn at a very early age to rub energetically directly over the site of an acute pain to reduce the noxious sensation. In the case of a more chronic discomfort from aching, 'knotted' muscle we tend to massage the local tissues more deeply and vigorously, even though doing so may temporarily exacerbate the discomfort. This is likely to be conditioned behaviour resulting from the analgesic effect of somatic sensory stimulation. With the development of stone tools it is easy to hypothesize a progression of therapeutic techniques which resulted ultimately in piercing the skin and muscle at a site of chronic pain. It may be that the success in treating myofascial pain by piercing the body at the site of tenderness encouraged the practice. In some parts of the world people developed superficial techniques of scratching or cauterizing the skin, whereas in the Far and Middle East acupuncture developed.

The development of acupuncture points probably resulted from clinical observation that certain places in the body were more likely to harbour tender points than others and that treating these points by pressure or piercing could relieve pain and various other non-painful symptoms. Consistent patterns of pain referral from myofascial trigger points and the relief resulting from needling these and other muscle points would have led them to make links between some of the points. Radiation patterns of painful medical conditions such as sciatica, other radiculopathies and possibly the consistent rashes of herpes zoster would have added to the impression that the established points were connected. The way light reflects off the oiled or moist surface of the body may also have had an influence on the way connections between points were perceived (A.J.R. MacDonald, personal communication).

These hypotheses by no means explain the location of all acupuncture points, nor the paths of all the meridians, but there is clearly considerable overlap between myofascial trigger points and acupuncture points (Melzack *et al.*, 1977) and between trigger point pain referral patterns and meridians (Figure 2.1).

The ancient Chinese physicians initially developed the system of acupuncture within the philosophical and cultural framework of Taoism, a system that follows the 'wu-wei'. That means to submit to the spontaneous impulses of one's own essential nature and to achieve unity with the Tao ('way'), the underlying pattern of the universe, an abstract force responsible for creation, interconnectedness, change and develop-

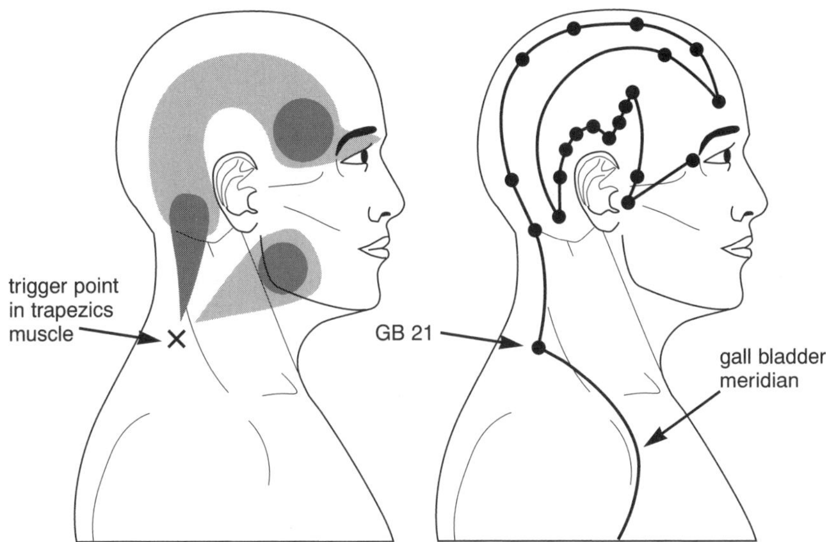

Figure 2.1 Trigger point pain referral patterns and meridians.

ment in all things. This 'go with the flow' philosophy is very appealing to people who feel trapped in the high-pressure environment of the west, which partly explains the increasing popularity of therapies like acupuncture which are perceived to go 'back to nature'.

Central to the beliefs of the Chinese physician was the existence of qi ('chi') or vital energy. This idea of vital energy may have derived from something as simple as observation of the life to death cycle, which is apparent throughout nature. More specifically it was noted that breathing and the intake of food were both necessary to maintain vital energy or life. But these two external factors were not all that was required for life and health, and the idea of innate energy was included. The possible contribution of a metaphysical dimension to the 'life force' is beyond the remit of this book and the subject of eternal debate. Undoubtedly any treatment has effects on both mind and body and this chapter is devoted to the effects that have been studied.

On a more mundane and tangible level, if one combines the philosophical idea of vital energy with the clinical observation of trigger points, tender points and pain referral patterns, it does not seem unreasonable for the ancients to have formed the idea that vital energy flows from point to point along channels in the body. The development of symptoms such as pain would lead the physician to examine along the channels for a blockage of energy flow. Discovery of a particularly tender point, palpation of which may have caused the subject to jump and shout 'ah shi' (Oh yes), clearly indicated the site of 'blockage'. Needling this point, recognized today as a myofascial trigger point, would frequently have resulted in decrease in tenderness of the point and resolution of the symptoms, powerfully reinforcing the idea that the blockage of energy flow had resolved.

Once this concept of energy flow in channels had been established, it evolved in complexity to explain many of the subsequent observations made from a myriad of clinical signs and symptoms. As this complexity grew, and in the absence of the modern scientific method, which systematically tests and discards unsupported hypotheses, the system of medicine probably became unwieldy. Thus when attempting to reinterpret the traditional ideas with a western perspective, 'the boundaries between concrete observations and the extrapolations are not always clear' (Beyens, 1998).

The sense of a universal duality in the interrelationship between all things is a concept that was shared by several cultures. The Chinese referred to yin and yang as the natural polarity in all things created by the Tao and applied the idea to energy flow in the body in a systematic way. Yin and yang were thought of as opposing forces of nature which complement each other in a dynamic process. It is easy to apply such a theory of opposites (light and dark, positive and negative, active and inactive) to the interpretation of basic clinical observation. Indeed the concept of two opposing yet interacting forces that are balanced in health has such flexibility that it can be applied to many systems in the body. Analogies can be made with the western nineteenth century theory of homeostasis proposed by Claude Bernard, which is widely supported by physiological research, or the view of contemporary epidemiologists who describe illness as being caused by a loss of equilibrium in the simultaneous interaction of host, agent and environment (Itoh and Lee, 1971). However, such flexibility of interpretation leads one to question the actual value of such a concept to the practising physician, despite its use to the philosopher.

No detailed anatomical studies were undertaken in China until the present century, so it is not at all surprising that the correlations made between organs and their attributed functions are wildly inaccurate in comparison with what we understand today in medical science. The heart in TCA is the principal organ that governs mental and higher conscious activities. Physicians probably observed the cardiac response to emotion, and concluded that the 'heart controls the mind'. In physiological terms the heart does not exert control over the 'mind', but reacts to demands from elsewhere and the overall control of the autonomic nervous system. In a similar way, many valid clinical observations must have been understandably misinterpreted, and became incorporated in traditional theory. Contrary evidence has only accrued latterly, nearly 2000 years after TCA had become established in practice. Proponents of TCA argue that the discipline is not static, but constantly evolving; however, the value of such evolution is questionable if it is not tested by scientific principles and discoveries.

Tongue and pulse diagnosis probably became prominent as a result of the influence of Confucianism when the physician's access to the whole body was limited by cultural mores. To date there is no evidence to support the contention that useful diagnostic information can be derived from pulse diagnosis over and above orthodox clinical examination (Vincent, 1992).

We know only too well from our history in the west that social, political and religious influences have affected the freedom of clinicians to develop and change practice. The courageous few who stood against the flow of popular opinion often paid a high price for promoting their ideas. Such factors clearly influenced the development of TCA and go some way to explaining why its fundamental concepts have remained unchallenged until quite recently. The practice of puncturing the body as a form of therapy has probably continued in some form for thousands of years, but Beyens (1998) cautions that 'The ancientness of acupuncture does not justify the systematic acceptance of the Chinese vision of this particular technique'. Nevertheless, any treatment which has survived for over 2000 years of battles, wars and successive dynasties is worthy of serious consideration.

Western acupuncture practice

The principal difference between a traditional eastern and western scientific acupuncture approach is the method of diagnosis and the relentless pursuit of a scientific rationale for treatment.

Central to western medicine as practised widely across the world, both east and west, is the formulation of a diagnosis based on best current practice. It involves taking a clinical history, making a clinical examination of the whole patient, or the relevant system, and interpreting the results of appropriate investigations. This leads to the initial formulation of a differential followed ideally by a definitive diagnosis, although it should be remembered that a definitive diagnosis may only result from an ongoing process of reassessment during the treatment process.

When a diagnosis is made, a range of therapeutic options is available depending on resources and the most suitable should be chosen for the patient, whether medication, surgery, referral to another specialist, or a non-pharmacological therapy. Acupuncture may be an appropriate form of therapy for any presenting patient, but there are circumstances in which it may not. For example, acupuncture is unethical treatment for bacterial meningitis where antibiotic treatment is available. Acupuncture is inappropriate for sensorineural deafness, because it has been shown to have no effect (Eisenberg *et al.*, 1974; Madell, 1975; Taub, 1975; Yarnell *et al.*, 1976). Acupuncture is inappropriate for undiagnosed cancer, because it can alleviate symptoms (Thompson and Filshie, 1997) and hence could mask its presence or delay its diagnosis. However, in the absence of suitable conventional therapy, acupuncture could be useful in a range of conditions, and may result in some alleviation of symptoms. There are 'grey' areas of practice, where there is some evidence for the efficacy of acupuncture; for example, it may be used for amoebic dysentery (Cheng *et al..*, 1979; Qiu *et al.*, 1979; Zhang *et al.*, 1979), although conventional opinion does not recommend acupuncture for this indication.

Another reason for preferring a therapy is that it may be much safer than the alternatives. Recently, Lazarou *et al.* (1998) have shown that drugs are between the fourth and sixth leading cause for deaths in the USA. So it is hardly surprising that there is unprecedented interest in non-drug treatment worldwide. Acupuncture is not without potential side-effects (see Chapter 6), but as Ernst points out (E. Ernst, personal communication), 'The side effects of acupuncture are "dimensions" less than those of drugs'.

A western approach to acupuncture would not be possible without the many notable researchers who have begun to examine in greater detail neurophysiological and neuropharmacological mechanisms. Acupuncture has only begun to gain any acceptance in conventional medical circles since the discovery of transferable analgesia from treated to untreated animals by cross circulation of blood and cerebrospinal fluid. Segmental sensory and autonomic modulation and a huge cast of neurophysiological players, including enkephalins, endorphins, dynorphins, serotonin, oxytocin, CGRP (calcitonin gene-related peptide), NGF (nerve growth factor), CCK (cholecystokinin) and many more are contributing to our deeper understanding of how acupuncture works. Contemporary knowledge about complex interactions between all these molecules and others possibly involved is likely to be fragmentary and incomplete. Most research into mechanisms has looked at limited neurophysiological events over short time spans. Further dynamic and metabolic imaging by MRI, and further PET scan initiatives after Jones *et al.* (1991) will be useful for future indirect assessments of function. Much research has explored experimental pain models that do not necessarily mimic disease in humans. Price *et al.* (1984) suggested that acupuncture may produce long-term analgesia which far outlives the duration of experimental pain relief in patients with back pain, although the design of the study did not allow for non-specific effects of needling.

Methods of treatment

There are many methods of practising acupuncture, possibly even as many variations in technique as there are acupuncturists, with subtle or great differences between individuals.

The methods range from a strict TCA approach based on meridian theory, with needle sensation strongly elicited at multiple sites, to an orthodox diagnostic approach followed by superficial brief needling. Felix Mann, an experienced, traditionally trained, pioneering acupuncture practitioner, has repeatedly challenged the traditional concepts and now no longer believes in the existence of discrete acupuncture points at all (Mann, 1992). The majority of medical acupuncture practitioners trained by eastern or western schools practise somewhere between these approaches, using a combination of trigger points, tender points, segmental points, and the most commonly used traditional points, often referred to as 'strong' points. Many use an eclectic approach (Campbell, 1998). The use of myofascial trigger points and segmental acupuncture points underpins the western approach to treatment, and both of these areas have sections of this chapter devoted to them.

Other acupuncture techniques in common use in the west include electroacupuncture and the use of semipermanent indwelling needles.

Transcutaneous electrical nerve stimulation (TENS) is often grouped with acupuncture as a complementary form of stimulation-produced analgesia, although it has a different mode of action. Microsystems such as auriculotherapy (Nogier, 1972; Oleson *et al.*, 1980) and scalp acupuncture (Yamamoto, 1989, 1998) have developed, and may rely on the rich innervation of the areas needled rather than from any hypothetical somatotopic representation of the whole body on these areas. Lewith and Vincent (1998) have, on the basis of sham controlled trials for smoking cessation, said that the specific point location may be unimportant in auriculoacupuncture for this indication.

As well as a great range in technique, there is also considerable variety in description of practice. Some western practitioners abandon the use of the term acupuncture altogether, partly on account of the prejudice they encounter from their orthodox colleagues. Gunn (1989) coined the term 'intramuscular stimulation', possibly more accurately describing the type of needle technique he employs; many pain clinics describe the use of 'dry needling', and some researchers, including Johansson *et al.* (1993), describe acupuncture as 'sensory stimulation' to overcome perceived publication bias.

Western-based acupuncture treatment

Acupuncture is used to treat painful and non-painful conditions. The painful conditions can be further classified as:

- Myofascial pain – where a trigger point approach to treatment predominates.
- Non-myofascial: nociceptive pain and visceral pain – which are best approached with segmental acupuncture.
- Neurogenic pain – where direct segmental stimulation may be effective, or may exacerbate symptoms, in which case an extra-segmental approach (using segments which are not hyperalgesic) may be used.
- Acute pain or surgical pain – when acupuncture may be used in addition to anaesthesia or sedation.

Non-painful conditions are more commonly treated with a local or segmental approach, or for generalized conditions a selection of well-known traditional points.

Empirically, many primary care physicians find an application for acupuncture in the management of a wide variety of musculoskeletal complaints. The incidence of musculoskeletal problems in primary care varies considerably, and is measured in several different ways. A recent survey of 6000 adults between the ages of 45 and 64 showed that 27% of females and 28% of males had suffered musculoskeletal pain in the previous month of at least 1 week's duration (Urwin *et al.*, 1999). The proportion of the population with chronic pain at any one time was estimated to be 11% in the UK (Bowsher *et al.*, 1991) and 14.4% in the USA (Magni *et al.*, 1990).

The Clinical Standards Advisory Group (1999) found that 86% of 122 pain clinics (chronic pain services) sampled, offer acupuncture as a modality of treatment. There appears to be a spectrum of disorder, from myofascial pain on the one hand to fibromyalgia on the other, with some overlapping features (McCain, 1993). So it seems that the primary myofascial complaints are both the most common, and the easiest to treat with acupuncture and similar techniques (see below).

Musculoskeletal pain is clearly a significant problem in both primary and secondary care, and it is likely that the efficacy of western acupuncture techniques in this area (trigger point and segmental acupuncture), when established, will be the key factor in the comprehensive acceptance and incorporation of acupuncture into western orthodox medicine. Therefore, the following two sections of this chapter have been devoted solely to a discussion of myofascial trigger points and segmental acupuncture.

Myofascial trigger points

Definition and history

A myofascial trigger point (TP), as defined by Travell and Simons (1983), is a hyperirritable locus within a taut band of skeletal muscle or its associated fascia. The TP is painful on compression and can exhibit a characteristic referral pattern of pain or autonomic dysfunction, and may also exhibit a jump sign and twitch response. The location of TPs often correlates precisely with that of acupuncture points (Melzack *et al.*, 1977), and their associated referral patterns sometimes describe a strikingly similar path to the meridian. This association is best illustrated by the TP often found in the upper free border of trapezius, precisely at the acupuncture point GB 21 (Figure 2.1).

Over the last century and a half, a number of different terms has been applied to the TP in the west, resulting in considerable confusion for the physician. Terms such as 'muscle callouses' (Froriep, 1843), 'muscular rheumatism' (Virchow, 1852), 'myitis chronica rheumatica' (Helleday, 1876), 'myogelosis' (Schade, 1921) and 'muscle hardenings' (Lange and Eversbusch, 1921) were the forerunners to the term 'fibrositis' which was introduced by Gowers in 1904. The latter term has survived in common use until surprisingly recently, considering that inflammation of connective tissue has never been consistently and reliably demonstrated in biopsy studies (Travell and Simons, 1983). Having noted the pain referral patterns described by some of his patients with tender muscle nodules, Kellgren (1938) investigated the pain referral patterns produced by injecting hypertonic saline into the muscles and other soft tissues of experimental subjects, and in true scientific spirit, subjected himself to many such procedures. Injecting into muscle he found that the resultant pain was more diffuse than when injecting into other soft tissues, and that as the stimulus intensified the pain pattern could spread over a wide area. Kellgren and his peers concluded that the distributions were generally segmental, but recognized that the pain must have a 'common path' in the central nervous system when several spinal segments were included. Investigation of muscle pain syndromes continued independently on three continents following Kellgren's work. Formerly from Poland, (Gutstein) Good (1951) continued his work in England. He described the patient's pain reaction that was later termed the 'jump sign', and he felt that the process responsible for 'myalgic spots' was a local constriction of blood vessels due to overactivity of the sympathetic nerves supplying them. The Australian Michael Kelly (1945) evolved the concept that 'fibrositis' was a functional neurological disturbance due to a local rheumatic process, with little or no local pathology, and a central nervous system reflex disturbance causing the referred pain. Travell, an American physician, devoted her career to the study of 'myofascial trigger points'. She initially emphasized the importance of the referral pattern from the TP, and postulated that any fibroblastic proliferation was secondary to a functional disorder, with pathological changes occurring only if the condition existed for a long time. She went on to develop the concept that the self-sustaining characteristic of TPs depended on a feedback mechanism between the TP and the central nervous system (Travell, 1976). Latterly she collaborated with Simons (Travell and Simons, 1983) to produce a very comprehensive manual covering the field of what is now popularly termed myofascial pain syndromes.

Incidence and identification

Trigger points appear to be a common source of pain and dysfunction in the community, although accurate estimates of the prevalence are not readily available. Cummings (personal observation) has observed that about 20% of consultations in UK general practice result from myofascial pain. Sola and colleagues found evidence of myofascial dysfunction, judged by the presence of latent TPs in the posterior shoulder girdle, in half of a group of 200 men and women aged 17–35 (Sola *et al.*, 1955). In estimating the prevalence of myofascial pain one must consider the reliability with which TPs can be detected between observers (interobserver) and in the same observer over time (intraobserver). Nice *et al.* (1993) found little evidence of interobserver reliability in identifying TPs, but Njoo and Van der Does (1995) and Gerwin *et al.* (1997) have subsequently demonstrated interobserver reliability, which was improved by a period of training in the latter case.

For some time investigators have been using pressure sensitive devices to aid identification of TPs, and each method has proved to be reliable (Reeves *et al.*, 1986; Delaney and McKee, 1993; Bendtsen *et al.*, 1994). Thermographic imaging has also been employed in the evaluation of TPs, and though the practicality of this technique in routine practice is questionable, it is interesting to note the observation of a reduction in temperature over a TP sensory referral area on compression of the TP (Kruse and Christiansen, 1992).

So it appears that sufficient training and the use of objective pressure measurement each allow us to reliably identify TPs in patients with myofascial pain compared with healthy controls. However, distinguishing the TPs of myofascial pain syndrome from the tender points of fibromyalgia has proved more of a challenge. Experts from both fields have found their examination skills unreliable (Wolfe *et al.*, 1992), and even the use of objective pressure measurement has been unhelpful

(Tunks *et al.*, 1995). On a practical level, the distinction between the two conditions is not often a clinical problem, when consideration is given to the history and the distribution of tender points. However, it may be useful to note that injecting TPs in patients with fibromyalgia and myofascial pain syndrome has been shown to cause significantly more postinjection soreness for a longer period of time than injecting TPs in patients without fibromyalgia (Hong and Hsueh, 1996).

Aetiology and classification

Travell and Simons (1983) put forward three causative factors responsible for the development of primary TPs: acute physical overload, overwork fatigue and chilling. They also describe secondary TPs developing as a result of some other pathological process or event.

TPs are either active, causing pain, or latent, resulting in weakness and restriction of movement of the affected muscle without pain. Active TPs are often associated with deep, dull, aching pain, which may be referred some distance. The referral pattern may be elicited by compression or needling of the TP. Hong *et al.* (1997) have recently found that the referral pattern of a TP is more frequently produced by TP injection than palpation, and that the frequency of occurrence of a referral pattern is significantly correlated with the pain intensity of the TP. Empirical evidence suggests that active TPs occur most commonly in the postural muscles of the neck, shoulder and hip girdle, and that middle-aged women are the most likely section of the population to seek treatment for myofascial pain (Travell and Simons, 1983). Bendtsen *et al.* (1996) have recently investigated the nociceptive process in the myofascial pain of patients with chronic tension-type headache as compared with healthy controls. They found that the relationship between pressure over a TP and the associated pain was linear, i.e. increments in pressure were proportional to the resulting increments in pain, whereas over normal muscle the relationship was non-linear; typically increments in pressure over normal muscle do not cause pain until a threshold is reached, when pain increases disproportionately. The authors postulate that myofascial pain is mediated by low-threshold mechanosensitive afferents projecting to sensitized dorsal horn neurones.

Neurophysiological evidence

Numerous biopsy studies have failed to demonstrate any specific histological features of the TP, although a study of single cell morphology has demonstrated a difference between muscle cells from patients with fibromyalgia and those with chronic myofascial pain (Jacobsen *et al.*, 1991). Gerwin (1994) notes that, despite years of clinical study, the pathophysiology of the TP has remained elusive, yet thanks to Hubbard and Berkoff (1993) there is now electromyographic evidence supporting the presence of at least a functional abnormality at the TP. There have been several negative electromyographic studies of TPs over the last 30 years, including one reported by Durette *et al.* (1991), but Hubbard and Berkoff (1993) have demonstrated increased electrical activity within an area of 1 or 2 mm around the TP relative to a normal area of the same muscle. This finding has been repeated in the UK by Ward (1996), who demonstrated spontaneous electrical activity in TPs at two locations which were also acupuncture points. Hubbard and Berkoff continued in cooperation with McNulty and Gervirtz (McNulty *et al.*, 1994) to show that a psychological stressor significantly increased the electrical activity of trapezius TPs compared with a non-stressful control task. So we now have a pathophysiological marker for the TP, and can see that it is influenced by stress, perhaps mediated by sympathetic tone.

Treatment of trigger points

It is likely that physical therapies have been used to treat myofascial pain for hundreds, if not thousands, of years. Around the world different communities have developed their own techniques, and even today TPs are approached in a variety of ways, ranging from simple muscle stretching manoeuvres (Travell and Simons, 1983; Lewit and Simons, 1984; Jaeger and Reeves, 1986) to ischaemic compression (Travell and Simons, 1983) which involves firm pressure being applied to the TP for about 1 minute. Such non-invasive techniques can be safely taught to patients suffering from myofascial pain syndromes, and can be especially useful if the condition follows a chronic relapsing course.

Clinical aspects of acupuncture treatment

As needling in the form of acupuncture has probably been applied to TPs for at least 3000 years, it is surprising that much of the recent research in this area has focused on TP injection techniques rather than acupuncture. Such techniques are sometimes referred to as 'wet needling', and the term 'dry needling' is applied to the use of the needle alone. When reference is made to dry needling it is important to differentiate between the use of a bevelled hypodermic needle, designed for injections, and the solid acupuncture needle. The former has a cutting edge and has the potential to cause considerably more tissue damage than the acupuncture needle, which separates fibres rather than cutting them. Moreover the diameter of hypodermic needles is considerably greater than that of acupuncture needles.

There is limited clinical research in this area of musculoskeletal therapy. However, wet and dry needling have been compared and appear to have similar efficacy in treating myofascial pain (Garvey *et al.*, 1989; Hong, 1994). Fine *et al.* (1988) have demonstrated a naloxone reversible effect in TP injections, suggesting a central opioid pathway is involved in the mechanism of action. This finding seems to support the contention that it is the needle rather than the injected substance that mediates the effect. Further support for this idea comes from studies which indicate that the nature of the injected substance does not significantly affect the efficacy of the technique; Tschopp and Gysin (1996) compared physiological saline with bupivacaine, and Wreje and Brorsson (1995) compared saline and sterile water. Some injected substances have proved to be more efficacious when compared to local anaesthetic: Frost (1986) used diclofenac – equivalent to a 50-mg intramuscular dose; and Cheshire *et al.* (1994) used botulinum toxin (type A).

Baldry (1996, 1998) elegantly describes clinical aspects of TP location and therapy, and Gunn (1997) uses a more invasive style of needling with a customized needle holder for intramuscular stimulation (IMS) to tender areas in shortened muscle.

Segmental acupuncture

'Segmental acupuncture' is the technique of needling an area innervated by the same spinal segment as the disordered structure under treatment. It has been practised since the earliest use of acupuncture therapies, though not by name or design. The use of 'local' points and 'Ah shi' points will almost inevitably involve treatment of the correct level in segmental terms. 'Distant' points are less likely to fall within the same segment. However, there are a number of examples of classical points which do, such as SP 6 (S2 myotome) for uterine problems.

The term segmental acupuncture has been used since Melzack and Wall (1965) described segmental pain modulation at the spinal dorsal horn in their 'Gate Control Theory', and it is now well established as a method of point selection by western medical practitioners.

Use of this technique requires determination of the segmental innervation of the area being treated and the somatic distribution of those segments as a target for needling. Each segment of the spinal cord innervates one or two areas of skin (dermatome), a section of paraxial as well as ventral or limb musculature (myotome), one or more areas of periosteum (sclerotome), and a portion of the viscera (viscerotome). This seems fairly straightforward, but there are a number of complexities and uncertainties to face:

- Precise segmental innervation in humans has not been established, and until recently knowledge has been based on clinical information derived from studies of denervation injuries documented in the earlier half of this century (*Gray's Anatomy*, 1995).
- Study of human embryology is useful, but differential rates of growth in the axial structures and the formation of limbs complicate segmental patterns, consequently dermatomes, myotomes and sclerotomes rarely overlap.
- Sympathetic efferent innervation of the soma originates in segments some distance from those supplying the bulk of the somatic outflow.

Clearly, neural tracer studies cannot be performed in humans, so in the last few years investigators have used various techniques in an attempt to further our knowledge of segmental innervation in humans; for example, opportunistic studies in patients undergoing selective posterior rhizotomy (Phillips and Park, 1991, 1993), needle electrophysiological studies (Ligouri *et al.*, 1992) and action potential magnetic field measurements (Epstein, 1993). These studies serve to confirm conventional ideas of segmental innervation, but perhaps add further uncertainty regarding the frequency of anomalous patterns.

In the last decade, neurophysiologists have come to appreciate that the spinal segment is considerably more than a relay station with the job of prioritizing incoming information. The discovery that afferent nerves have a secretory role in the periphery has resulted in a better understanding of the ways in which anatomically distinct areas of the same segment may influence each other. Manual therapists of various disciplines have claimed to be able to influence distant parts of the body, and even visceral function, by spinal manipulation (Picalov and Kharin, 1994). Formerly this claim seemed somewhat ridiculous to people trained in medical science, but now it is more credible that under some circumstances such indirect influence is possible. The practice of traditional acupuncture has not been so clearly orientated to segmental relations, but more of its elements are understandable in the light of such influences. Beckering and van Bussel (1998) have produced a most interesting and elaborate theory that relies on extensive segmental interrelationships. The most courageous links they make are termed 'secondary segmental relations', and refer to the sympathetic supply to the soma. They propose three distinct grey columns running in parallel in the intermediate horn of the thoracolumbar spinal cord, responsible for sympathetic innervation of the viscera, the somatic thorax and abdomen, and the head and limbs. The latter column is proposed as follows: C8 to T4 to the head and neck; T5 to T9 to the upper limb; T10 to L2 to the lower limb. Perhaps the most contentious of these is the sympathetic supply to the upper limb. *Gray's Anatomy* (1995) states that this is from T2 to T5, and Koizumi and McC Brooks (1984) cover both options proposing T2 to T9. Nevertheless the potential segmental interrelationships are clearly far wider than one may at first appreciate. It is important to realize that the sympathetic nervous system is not a discrete system but an integral part of the whole, and can exert an influence on every part of the body. Equally, stimulation of any part of the body can modify sympathetic activity (Sato and Schmidt, 1973). Acupuncture-like stimulation in rats has been shown to cause a temporary increase in sympathetic tone, followed by a more prolonged depression (Yao, 1993), and in regional terms segmental as opposed to non-segmental stimulation appears to have a more potent effect on this sympathetic modulation (Sato *et al.*, 1992).

Clinical acupuncture research

Some of the difficulties in acupuncture trial methodology are discussed here. Lewith and Vincent (1998) repeat the two questions which are of fundamental importance: first, does acupuncture have a beneficial effect on any disease or disorder, and second, is this effect due to the needle or the placebo effect. They rightly state that the most urgent task is to establish a unanimously agreed methodology for evaluation of these questions. The problems of dose, controls and rigorous trial design will be addressed here.

Dose of acupuncture

Ideally, there should be collective agreement on best practice for a given condition, but to date there is no real consensus and little or no evidence regarding the dose of acupuncture. In addition to the complex business of point selection, there are a large number of other variables to consider, such as the number of needles per treatment, the diameter of each needle, the depth of stimulation; subcutaneous, intramuscular or periosteal, and the type of stimulation or agitation of needles, electrical or various manual techniques, and the duration of needling.

There is a wide variation in the acupuncture 'dose' which could affect the response. Early meta-analyses of acupuncture have not adequately described these essential data, largely because treatment details are poorly recorded in many papers (Ter Reit *et al.*, 1990a, 1990b; Kleijnen *et al.*, 1991; Patel *et al.*, 1989). This leaves the potential for incorrect conclusions to be reached when incompatible 'doses' of treatment have been given to acupuncture sites with different innervation.

In a meta-analysis of acupuncture treatment for back pain, Ernst and White (1998) have attempted to address the problem of comparable 'dose' by incorporating a blinded assessment of the quality of acupuncture given, described by White and Ernst (1998). Even in this study, insufficient account was taken of the classification of pain, for example, neurogenic or nociceptive, as recommended by Thomas (1995), but this was inevitable on account of insufficient information in the original reports.

One systematic review in which the 'dose' in different studies was probably comparable was on treatment of nausea and vomiting (Vickers, 1996). Twenty-seven out of 29 trials of acupuncture at PC 6 showed acupuncture to be significantly superior to placebo. In the remaining four trials, acupuncture stimulation was given under anaesthesia, and proved to be equal or inferior to the control treatment. In 12 of the high quality trials when it was not given under anaesthesia, 11 involving 1932 patients showed the positive effect of PC 6 treatment. The PC 6 single-point treatment allowed trial design to be simplified. The condition allowed manageable follow-up times and the hard objective outcome measure of vomiting, although nausea is clearly subjective. The conditions it was used for were nausea and vomiting due to surgery, cancer chemotherapy or pregnancy. PC 6 was treated either with needles (stimulated manually or electrically) or with acupressure. Control groups received either no intervention, local anaesthesia, dummy point stimulation, placebo 'seabands' or inactive TENS machines. Trials were conducted by eight principal investigators in seven different sites using different forms of PC 6 stimulation. Some problems in trial methodology for nausea and vomiting have been discussed by McMillan (1998).

The 'dose' was probably comparable in these single-point acupuncture treatment trials and the trials were akin to comparing 'apples with apples' despite the considerable variation in choice of controls. By contrast, acupuncture trials for many different forms of headache reviewed by Hester (1998) showed a wide variety of treatment schedules, treatment times from 2 minutes to 20 minutes, a wide variety of control procedures, and follow-up periods ranging from 1 day to 2 years. Not surprisingly there were widely conflicting results. This is a clear case of comparing 'apples with pears', and this approach has been taken by Ter Riet *et al.* (1990a) comparing different clinical pain problems with different treatment schedules, controls and follow up, with predictably conflicting results. Such reviews can only really address the quality of the studies performed, rather than give any meaningful measure of efficacy.

Drug trials are based on dose–response studies for tightly controlled specific indications and show considerable pharmacokinetic variation in response. Acupuncture studies are not, although for experimental pain, Brockhaus and Elger (1990) have elegantly shown a population distribution graph for the analgesic response to needling at LI14 compared with placebo point stimulation and showed a range from non-responders to high responders for active treatment in volunteers.

Controls

The methodological difficulties and challenges in finding suitably acceptable controls for acupuncture trials has probably been the major obstruction to the acceptance of this technique by the conventional medical community. Regrettably, the bulk of the acupuncture literature, which is of Chinese origin, has been dominated by uncontrolled case series in which an apparently homogeneous group of patients is not clearly defined by inclusion and exclusion criteria. Research is rarely prospective and it is not clear from the reporting whether consecutive subjects or selected subjects are recruited. A lack of control groups introduces bias and it is also rare to find an independent observer assessing the outcome. In much of the literature from China, outcome measures are vague, with results expressed in groups referred to as 'cured', 'greatly improved' and 'slightly improved'. Statistical analysis is frequently absent.

Table 2.1 includes a number of possible choices of control group, both tested and untested, which will briefly be described here.

1. No treatment or 'waiting list' control

The use of a delayed treatment control group is considered ethically justifiable in trials of chronic, stable conditions, for example for chronic low back pain and neck pain (Coan *et al.*, 1980, 1982), and for knee pain (Christensen *et al.*, 1992). Differentiating between the specific and non-specific effects of acupuncture cannot be addressed using this type of trial.

2. Comparison with alternative treatment or standard care

These trials require acupuncture to be at least as good as standard care to establish its efficacy, and have the ethical advantage of treating all patients in the study. Patients with renal colic given acupuncture had a more rapid onset of analgesia, no side-effects and achieved similar pain relief as those given standard analgesic treatment (Lee *et al.*, 1992). The observational study, followed by a comparison with standard treatment, and then the addition of a third control group, is well illustrated by List and Helkimo (1987, 1992, 1993). They treated chronic facial pain with acupuncture in a pilot study of ten patients (1987), followed by a study comparing acupuncture to standard treatment (1992), and subsequently performed a three arm trial including a control group (1993). The latter

Table 2.1 Possible control groups

	Group	
1	waiting list	
2	alternative treatment or comparison with standard care	
3	invasive minimal sham acupuncture	at active treatment site away from active treatment site in same segment away from active treatment site in different segment away from active treatment site in distant segment
4	invasive standard stimulation sham acupuncture	away from active site in same segment away from active site in different segment away from active site in distant segment
5	non-invasive sham acupuncture	at active site away from active site
6	inactivated TENS	
7	laser treatment – active laser treatment – inactive	
8	transcutaneous spinal electroanalgesia (TSE)	active inactive
9	local anaesthetic (LA) prior to needling	LA injection followed by standard needling topical LA followed by standard needling
10	within-patient crossover with minimal acupressure	'dummy' semi-permanent press needle
11	multiple arms	different active or control therapy in each arm standard orthodox treatment plus active or control acupuncture in each arm
12	treatment rotation	rotation of a number of different treatments including a control, with a choice for the final treatment

trial showed the superiority of acupuncture and standard treatment over the control. When acupuncture was compared with oxybutynin treatment for patients with low compliant bladder problems, the acupuncture group experienced fewer side-effects and greater help with nocturia (Kelleher *et al.*, 1994). Again the non-specific effects of acupuncture are not addressed with these studies.

Acupuncture plus best standard treatment proved superior to standard treatment alone for patients with acute hemiplegic stroke (Johansson *et al.*, 1993). The acupuncture group showed greater improvements in balance, mobility, activities of daily living, and quality of life, and reduced duration of inpatient stay and rehabilitation costs. Similarly, a greater percentage of patients treated with acupuncture and physical therapy for low back pain returned to work compared with those who only received physical therapy (Gunn *et al.*, 1980).

Acupuncture can also be compared with standard treatment in 'double-dummy' designs. For example, Clavel-Chapelon *et al.* (1992) compared acupuncture and nicotine gum in a 2 × 2 factorial design, and Hesse *et al.* (1994) compared acupuncture plus sham metoprolol with sham acupuncture plus metoprolol.

3 & 4. Invasive sham acupuncture controls

A considerable variety of control needling techniques are available using needling at non-points or inappropriate points either intra- or extrasegmentally, or superficial needling at non-points intra- or extrasegmentally or at the correct points.

Superficial acupuncture with minimal stimulation, which can be assumed to trigger most of the non-specific effects of needling and may minimize the specific effects, was chosen in studies of acupuncture for facial pain (Hansen and Hansen, 1993), migraine (Vincent, 1989), fibromyalgia (Deluze *et al.*, 1992) and xerostomia (Blom *et al.*, 1992). Non-point acupuncture over the patella has been favoured by some investigators as a sham needling proceedure (Jobst *et al.*, 1986; Williamson *et al.*, 1996).

5. Non-invasive sham acupuncture controls

A non-acupuncture placebo treatment must be devised so that it is both credible and non-invasive (Vincent and Lewith, 1995; Lewith and Vincent, 1996), and the use of the credibility rating method described by Borkovec and Nau (1972) is recommended (Vincent, 1990).

Credible non-invasive needling techniques include a pencil-like probe (Molsberger and Hille, 1994), light tapping on skin with an introducer (Lao *et al.*, 1995), or a blunted cocktail stick tapped through an introducer. (White *et al.*, 1996). Some trials have included less credible placebos, such as rubbing needles against the skin (Borglum-Jensen *et al.*, 1979) and gluing needles to the skin (Gallacchi *et al.*, 1981).

6. Inactivated TENS

'Dummy' or inactive TENS has been used for low back pain with a 'hi-tech' appearance – using a large device with a number of flashing lights, in an attempt to maximize the expectation of efficacy in the subjects (MacDonald *et al.*, 1983). Inactive TENS has also been used for neck pain (Petrie and Langley, 1983), and Dowson *et al.* (1985) found it to be as credible as acupuncture when used as a control.

7 & 8. Laser therapy and transcutaneous spinal electroanalgesia (TSE)

These therapies have the advantage that, whether active or inactive, they cannot be felt by the patient. The operator may also be unaware of whether the instrument is active, and therefore true double-blind studies can be performed. Laser has the added advantage that it can be used at standard acupuncture points. Inactive TENS, laser and TSE may not adequately control for the non-specific effects of needling, whereas they may successfully control for the other non-specific effects of acupuncture.

9. Local anaesthetic prior to needling

Local anaesthetic (LA) injections prior to needling have been shown to block both the analgesic effects of acupuncture (Chiang *et al.*, 1973) and the antiemetic effects (Dundee, Ghaly, 1991). Local anaesthetic at ST 36 failed to block the effect of electroacupuncture (EA) on gastric acid secretion (Tougas *et al.*, 1992). However, in this study the local anaesthetic injections also failed to block all sensation, and may have been incomplete.

If the absorption characteristics of topical anaesthetics for the skin (LA cream) can be improved, inactive LA cream plus real needling versus active LA cream plus real needling may be a credible design which would take account of the non-specific effects of needling.

10. Within-patient crossover of standard treatment versus minimal acupressure

A dummy semi-permanent press needle has been designed to use in 'within-patient crossover' studies which need the semi-permanent needles in situ as the active treatment (J. Filshie, own design). This has the advantages of using the same site, looking identical to the patient and observer, and exerting minimal or no specific acupressure effect.

11. Multiple arms

Multiple arms have been used in studies on the efficacy of acupuncture. For example, Helms (1987) used standard acupuncture for dysmenorrhoea versus a sham needling procedure versus a standard control group versus a 'visitation' control group in order to try and ascertain which aspects were responsible for relief of pain.

12. Treatment rotation

Thomas *et al.* (1995) in another study on dysmenorrhoea used four types of acupuncture and three types of TENS with a patient crossover technique. Patients chose their preferred mode of stimulation in the last phase of the trial. In a similarly designed study on the treatment of back pain, Thomas and Lundeberg (1994) showed that low-frequency EA may have a prolonged effect on reducing pain compared with normal acupuncture and high-frequency EA.

In order to determine the specific effects of acupuncture as well as to compare it with standard care, a three armed trial design of active acupuncture treatment versus minimal/sham acupuncture versus best standard treatment should be used. Sample size should be adequate to ensure that any real differences reach statistical significance. It would also be advantageous to accommodate an individualized approach to the treatment, as the use of formula-based treatment in most clinical trials to date may have contributed to under evaluation of the efficacy of acupuncture treatment. However, individualized treatments do not exclude bias in therapist–subject interaction with active and control groups. This may be minimized by standardized interaction. Space does not permit more than a short section on clinical trials in this chapter. For a detailed review of the value of acupuncture in a wide range of clinical areas, refer to Chapter 5 of this book or *Medical Acupuncture, A Western Scientific Approach* (Filshie and White, 1998).

Design, conduct, reporting of trials

Good trial design aims to exclude bias, which can affect the outcome of trials in many ways (Sackett 1979). The study described below presents many features of a trial that gives a definitive answer to a clinically relevant question.

Kelleher *et al.* (1994) compared acupuncture with conventional optimal treatment (oxybutynin) in a prospective randomized controlled trial of 39 women with idiopathic low compliance with urge incontinence, frequency and nocturia. All patients completed a detailed urinary symptom diary, a symptom visual analogue scale and a urinary diary prior to objective urodynamic investigations. All patients had a diagnosis of low compliance (a tonic detrusor pressure rise of >15 cmH_2O for <500 ml during cystometry). Six-weekly treatments were given with minimal interaction between patient and acupuncturist. Six-weekly visits were also given to the oxybutynin group, to control for the attention given to the acupuncture group. The oxybutynin group received a dose of 5 mg b.d. The acupuncture points used were BL 23, BL 28 and two further lumbar paravertebral and four sacral segmental points, plus SP 6 and ST 36 bilaterally and CV 3.

Symptoms of urgency and frequency were significantly improved by both treatments and nocturia by acupuncture. Greater benefit was found at 6 weeks than at 3 weeks. Urge incontinence did not improve in either group; however, bladder compliance improved in both. Although there were no significant differences between the groups, the side-effect profile was considerably better in the acupuncture group, with three women withdrawing from the study due to side-effects in the oxybutynin group. At 3 months, eight out of 20 in the acupuncture group were symptom free and four had slight urgency but did not require treatment, while seven out of 19 were symptom free on oxybutynin. Thus, in the only study comparing acupuncture with conventional treatment, acupuncture was found to be comparable in effectiveness but with significantly fewer side-effects. Mechanisms of action need further elucidation but enkephalinergic nerves have been demonstrated in smooth muscle strips by Alm *et al.* (1981). Human detrusor muscle has been shown to be sensitive to methionine and leucine enkephalins *in vitro* by inhibiting evoked detrusor contractions (Klarskov, 1987). This suggests a presynaptic inhibitory activity of enkephalins on the bladder. Opioid antagonism with naloxone enhances detrusor activity in cats (Roppolo *et al.*, 1983), rats (Dray *et al.*, 1984) and humans (Murray and Feneley, 1982; Murray, 1983). This lends support to the endogenous opioid theory of acupuncture and it seems likely that segmental modulation of autonomic reflexes is a key mechanism (Sato *et al.*, 1992).

The general principles applicable to acupuncture trial design were listed by Ter Riet *et al.* (1990a) as quality criteria. These have been combined with details from *Good Clinical Practice for Trials* (Committee for Proprietary Medicinal Products Working Party on Efficacy of Medicinal Products, 1990) to create a list of important features for trial design, conduct and reporting (Table 2.2).

The placebo effect

There are many prejudices in life, and some people are 'acupuncturist'! These people say that the effect of acupuncture is 'only' due to the 'placebo' effect. The placebo effect or the non-specific effect of treatment can be very powerful, and there is wide current debate about both its precise definition and the nature of the response (Richardson, 1990; Roberts *et al.*, 1993; Wall, 1994; Ernst and Resch, 1995; Benson, 1996).

As already mentioned, the placebo effect appears to evoke responses by increasing endogenous opioids (Levine *et al.*, 1979). A recent systematic review (Ter Riet *et al.*, 1998) has confirmed that the placebo effect is mediated via endogenous opioids, and Hersh *et al.* (1993) have shown a naltrexone reversible analgesic effect mediated by a placebo treatment. Apparently we may have the challenging scenario in which both acupuncture and placebo treatments have common pathways in analgesia, so how can we possibly delineate one from the other? Thomas (1997), having identified this problem, tried to investigate the differences more closely by re-examining a study he performed in 1991 with Eriksson

Table 2.2 Some important features of trial design, conduct and reporting including those derived from Ter Riet *et al.* (1990) and Good Clinical Practice (Committee for Proprietary Medicinal Products (CPMP) Working Party on Efficacy of Medicinal Products, 1990)

Thorough literature review
Ethics approval and protection of subjects
Clear research question
Written protocol
Adequate choice and application of acupuncture treatment
Sample size and power calculation
Informed consent
Explicit method of recruitment of homogeneous sample
Specified inclusion and exclusion criteria
Baseline data for comparison
Prestratification if appropriate
Appropriate method of randomization and concealment
Choice of valid outcome measures
Blinded independent observer
Adequate follow-up period
Correct method of data collection, storage and handling
Appropriate statistical analysis
Monitoring of trial conduct
Publication of full final report
Include adequate description of acupuncture procedure
Include report of adverse events
Include adequate information for reader to do inferential statistics

and Lundeberg on patients with neck pain treated by either real acupuncture, superficial acupuncture, diazepam or dummy diazepam using a crossover protocol (Thomas *et al.*, 1991). The outcome showed significant reduction in both sensory and affective components of pain in all groups except the group that received dummy diazepam. This indicates that sham acupuncture was more effective than a placebo tablet. However, it cannot be concluded that the difference was due to a specific effect of the sham acupuncture. Sham acupuncture may simply be a more effective placebo. The truth is likely to be somewhere between these two positions, and this partly calls into question the use of sham or minimal acupuncture in trials. However, the sample size may have been inadequate to produce a definitive answer.

The therapeutic response depends on the complicated interaction of patient factors and expectations with therapist factors and his or her expectations, and treatment factors, including the specific and non-specific effects of the treatment. It is the responsibility of future researchers to overcome current methodological problems and prove or disprove the beneficial effects of acupuncture, although the authors of this chapter do at present have a slight bias in favour of the specific efficacy of acupuncture!

Attitudes to acupuncture are thought to influence the outcome of treatment. Levine *et al.* (1976) have shown that patients with high initial anxiety and depression scores have significantly more relief than patients with low scores. Similarly, Berlin *et al.* (1975) showed that patients with a higher level of anxiety gained a greater reduction in pain after treatment. Katz *et al.* (1974) have shown a positive correlation between hypnotic susceptibility and acupuncture analgesia in volunteers. In another study of acupuncture for chronic shoulder pain, however, that was specifically designed to test placebo effects and hypnotic susceptibility, Moore and Berk (1976) failed to show a real difference of effect when acupuncture was given in either a positive or an extraordinarily negative setting. A more recent study by Collier *et al.* (1995) showed no difference in attitudes to acupuncture and knowledge of acupuncture response between the 55% who were responders and the non-responders, and found a negative correlation between the acupuncture response and the trait of anxiety.

Attitudes to treatment in the clinical trial context are potentially changed subtly or greatly from a situation of reasonable contact between patient and therapist, to one of minimal contact. For example, contact between patient and therapist was artificially restricted in the trial of Kelleher *et al.* (1994); better results may have been obtained if the contact was more realistic.

The future

Acupuncture has survived thousands of years of clinical use and is only recently exciting clinical research interest. The intense conservatism and robust scepticism of conventional medical minds are a filter against outrageous claims, but can be frustrating when they demand more proof of efficacy than many conventional treatments in current daily use can boast.

Considerable progress could be made in the field of acupuncture with collective collaboration over trial design and methodology between major researchers world-wide. There is an urgency about organizing this as too much time has been spent by lone enthusiasts and inexperienced research teams, who may have repeated previous errors made by academics unfamiliar with the subject (Hayhoe, 1998).

Although this chapter has emphasized trigger point and segmental approaches to acupuncture, there are many observations from traditional acupuncture that cannot be explained in this way. For example, PC 6 is neither a trigger point, nor is it tender in nausea, nor is it a segmental point for the stomach: yet the evidence for its efficacy in nausea and vomiting is compelling (Vickers, 1996).

Little progress with studies can be made without considerable funding from government or charitable research trusts. One problem common to many potential researchers is that of 'invisible' literature in journals which are not accessible by simple Medline or Cochrane searches. For example, one of the better articles on the use of acupuncture for menopausal symptoms by Wyon *et al.* (1995) is difficult to find by searches of the conventional databases. Even if the quality of the publications is not perfect, access to previous findings would reduce unnecessary duplication of effort. A further international acupuncture journal to attract articles from across the world away from 'invisible' society journals would be one possible way forward, and negotiations are underway to deliver this (Hayhoe, 1998).

Further funding is necessary to perform cost–benefit analyses of different aspects of care, particularly in primary care, where early interaction within the first few months might reduce secondary referrals and hence help shift the burden of care from the high cost secondary care environment. These studies should include outcome measures of quality of life and activities of daily living in addition to specific disease-related parameters.

Anaesthetics is a particularly scientific specialty within medicine and yet the best clinical anaesthetists marry the science of the subject with the art of delivery. The same is possibly true of acupuncture. Although there is a fashion at present for evidence-based medicine, leaning heavily on meta-analyses and systematic reviews, Sir Douglas Black (1998) stresses 'the importance of the prior intellectual analysis of the problem, be it clinical or organisational in such a way was to define the type of evidence that is going to be relevant', and comments on the fact that medicine in general is both a science and an art. We should turn our emphasis to getting medicine-based evidence as well as evidence-based medicine (Knottnerus and Dinant, 1997), and over the next 50 years it is to be hoped that we can accomplish this objective for acupuncture.

Perhaps even one day it is possible that we shall be able to stimulate specific beneficial neurotransmitters non-invasively, and that needling itself could become obsolete.

References

Alm, P., Alumets, J., Hakanson, R. *et al.* (1981). Enkephalin immunoreactive nerve fibres in the feline genitourinary tract. *Histochemistry*, **72,** 351–355.

Baldry, P. E. (1996). *Acupuncture, Trigger Points and Musculo-Skeletal Pain*, 2nd edn. Edinburgh: Churchill Livingstone.

Baldry, P. E. (1998). Trigger point acupuncture. In *Medical Acupuncture, A Western Scientific Approach* (J. Filshie and A. White, eds), pp. 33–60. Edinburgh: Churchill Livingstone.

Beckering, R. and van Bussell, R. (1998). Segmental acupuncture. In *Medical Acupuncture, A Western Scientific Approach* (J. Filshie and A. White, eds), pp 105–135. Edinburgh: Churchill Livingstone.

Bendtsen, L., Jensen, R., Jensen, N. K. and Olesen, J. (1994). Muscle palpation with controlled finger pressure, new equipment for the study of tender myofascial tissues. *Pain*, **59,** 235–239.

Bendtsen, L., Jensen, R. and Olesen, J. (1996). Qualitatively altered nociception in chronic myofascial pain. *Pain*, **65,** 259–264.

Benson, H. (1996). *Timeless Healing. The Power and Biology of Belief.* London: Simon and Schuster.

Berlin, F., Bartlett, R., Black, J. (1975). Acupuncture and placebo. *Anaesthesiology*, **42,** 527–531.

Beyens, F. (1998). Reinterpretation of traditional concepts in acupuncture. In *Medical Acupuncture. A Western Scientific Approach* (J. Filshie and A. White, eds), pp. 391–407. Edinburgh: Churchill Livingstone.

Black, D. (1998). The limitations of evidence. *J. R. Coll. Physicians Lond.*, **32**(1), 23–26.

Blom, M., Dawidson, I. and Angmar-Mansson, B. (1992). The effect of acupuncture on salivary flow rates in patients with xerostomia. *Oral Surg. Oral Med. Oral Pathol.*, **73,** 293–298.

Borglum-Jensen, L., Melson, B. and Borglum-Jenson S. (1979). Effect of acupuncture on headache measured by reduction in number of attacks and use of drugs. *Scand. J. Dent. Res.*, **87,** 373–380.

Borkovec, T. D. and Nau, S. D. (1972). Credibility of analogue therapy rationales. *J. Behav. Ther. Exp. Psychol.*, **3**, 257–260.

Bowsher, D., Rigge, M. and Sopp. L. (1991). Prevalence of chronic pain in the British population. A telephone survey of 1037 households. *Pain Clin.*, **4,** 223–231.

Boyer, C. B. (1994) "Science," Microsoft ®Encarta. Copyright 1994 Microsoft Corporation. Copyright 1994 Funk and Wagnall's Corporation.

Brockhaus, A. and Elger, C. E. (1990). Hypalgesic efficacy of acupuncture on experimental pain in man. Comparison of laser acupuncture and needle acupuncture. *Pain*, **43,** 181–185.

Campbell, A. (1998). Methods of acupuncture. In *Medical Acupucture. A Western Scientific Approach* (J. Filshie and A. White, eds), pp. 19–32. Edinburgh: Churchill Livingstone.

Cheng, Z. C., Shi, P. F., Ji S. H. *et al.* (1979). *The Clinical Observation on the Acupuncture Treatment of Acute Bacillary Dysentery*. Beijing: People's Medical Publishing House 39.

Cheshire, W. P., Abashian, S. W. and Mann, J. D. (1994). Botulinum toxin in the treatment of myofascial pain syndrome. *Pain*, **59,** 65–69.

Chiang, C. Y., Chang, C. T., Chu, H. L. and Yang, L. F. (1973). Peripheral afferent pathway for acupuncture analgesia. *Sci. Sin.*, **16,** 210–217.

Christensen, B. V., Iuhl, I. U., Vilbek, H. *et al.* (1992). Acupuncture treatment of severe knee osteoarthritis, a long-term study. *Acta Anaesthesiol. Scand.*, **36,** 519–525.

Clavel-Chapelon, F., Paoletti, C. and Benhamou, S. (1992). A randomised 2 × 2 factorial design to evaluate different smoking cessation methods. *Rev. Epidemiol. Sante Publique*, **40,** 187–190.

Clinical Standards Advisory Group Report (1999). National Review of Pain Services and Standards. London: The Stationery Office.

Coan, R. M., Wong, G., Ku, S. L. *et al.* (1980). The acupuncture treatment of low back pain, a randomized controlled study. *Am. J. Chin. Med.*, **8,** 181–189.

Coan, R. M., Wong, G. and Coan, P. L. (1982). The acupuncture treatment of neck pain, a randomised controlled study. *Am. J. Chin. Med.*, **9**, 326–332.

Collier, S., Phillips, D., Camp, V. and Kirk, A. (1995). The influence of attitudes to acupuncture on the outcome of treatment. *Acupunct. Med.*, **13**, 74–77.

Committee for Proprietary Medicinal Products (CPMP) Working Party on Efficacy of Medicinal Products. (1990). Good clinical practice for trials on medicinal products in the European Community: EEC notes for guidance. *Pharmacology and Toxicology*, **67**, 361–372.

Delaney, G. A. and McKee, A. C. (1993). Inter- and intra-rater reliability of the pressure threshold meter in measurement of myofascial trigger point sensitivity. *Am. J. Phys. Med.*, **72**, 136–139.

Deluze, C., Bosia, L., Zirbs, A. *et al.* (1992). Electroacupuncture in fibromyalgia. Results of a controlled trial. *Br. Med. J.*, **305**, 1249–1252.

Dowson, D. I., Lewith, G. T. and Machin, D. (1985). The effects of acupuncture versus placebo in the treatment of headache. *Pain*, **21**, 35–42.

Dray, A., Metsch, R. and Davis, T. P. (1984). Endorphins and the central inhibition of urinary bladder motility. *Peptides*, **5**, 645–647.

Dundee, J. W. and Ghaly, G. (1991). Local anesthesia blocks the antiemetic action of P6 acupuncture. *Clin. Pharmacol. Ther.*, **50**, 78–80.

Durette, M. R., Rodriquez, A. A., Agre, J. C. and Silverman, J. L. (1991). Needle electromyographic evaluation of patients with myofascial or fibromyalgic pain. *Am. J. Phys. Med.*, **70**, 154–156.

Eisenberg, L., Taub, H. A. and DiCarlo, L. (1974). Acupuncture therapy of sensorineural deafness. Evaluation Study. *N. Y. State J. Med.*, **74**, 1942–1949.

Epstein, C. M. (1993). Magnetic mapping of human cervical nerve roots, variation in normal subjects. *Electroencephalogr. Clin. Neurophysiol. Electromyogr. Motor Control*, **89**, 145–153.

Ernst, E. and Resch, K-L (1995). Concept of true and perceived placebo effects. *Br. Med. J.*, **311**, 551–553.

Ernst, E. and White, A. R. (1998). Acupuncture for back pain, a meta-analysis of randomised controlled trials. *Arch. Int. Med.*, **158**, 2235–2241.

Filshie, J. and White, A. R. (1998). Acupuncture through the medical systems. In *Medical Acupuncture, A Western Scientific Approach* (J. Filshie and A. White, eds), pp. 225–294. Edinburgh: Churchill Livingstone.

Fine, P. G., Milano, R. and Hare, B. D. (1988). The effects of myofascial trigger point injections are naloxone reversible. *Pain*, **32**, 15–20.

Froriep, R. (1843). *Ein Beitrag zur Pathologie und Therapie des Rheumatismus*. Weimar.

Frost, A. (1986). Diclofenac versus lidocaine as injection therapy in myofascial pain. *Scand. J. Rheumatol.*, **15**, 153–156.

Gallacchi, G., Mueller, W., Plattner, G. R. and Schnorrenberger, C. C. (1981). Akupunktur- und Laserstrahlbehandlung beim Zervikal- und Lumbalsyndrom. *Schweiz. Med. Wochenschr.*, **111**, 1360–1366.

Garvey, T. A., Marks, M. R. and Weisel, S. W. (1989). A prospective, randomised, double-blind evaluation of trigger-point injection therapy for low-back pain. *Spine*, **14**, 962–964.

Gerwin, R. D. (1994). Neurobiology of the myofascial trigger point. *Baillière's Clin. Rheumatol.*, **8**, 747–762.

Gerwin, R. D., Shannon, S., Hong, C. Z. *et al.* (1997). Interrater reliability in myofascial trigger point examination. *Pain*, **69**, 65–73.

Good, M. G. (1951). Objective diagnosis and curability of nonarticular rheumatism. *Br. J. Phys. Med.*, **14**, 1–7.

Gowers, W. R. (1904). Lumbago, its lessons and analogues. *Br. Med. J.*, **1**, 117–121.

Gray's Anatomy (1995) 38th edn. London: Churchill Livingstone.

Gunn, C. C. (1989). *Treating Myofascial Pain, Intramuscular Stimulation (IMS) for Myofascial Pain Syndromes of Neuropathic Origin*. Seattle: University of Washington.

Gunn, C. C. (1997). *The Gunn Approach to the Treatment of Chronic Pain: IMS for myofascial pain of radiculopathic origin*. New York: Churchill Livingstone.

Gunn, C. C., Milbrandt, W. E., Little, A. S. and Mason, K. E. (1980). Dry needling of muscle motor points for chronic low back pain, a randomised clinical trial with long-term follow up. *Spine*, **5,** 279–291.

Han, J. S. (1987). *The Neurochemical Basis of Pain Relief by Acupuncture. A Collection of Papers 1973–1987.* Beijing Medical. Distributed by Acumedic.

Hansen, P. E. and Hansen, J. H. (1983). Acupuncture treatment of chronic facial pain – a controlled crossover trial. *Headache*, **23,** 66–69.

Hayhoe, S. (1998). The future. In *Medical Acupuncture. A Western Scientific Approach* (J. Filshie and A. White, eds), pp. 409–414. Edinburgh: Churchill Livingstone.

Helleday, U. (1876). Om myitis chronica (rheumatica). Et bidrag till dess diagnostik och behandling. *Nord. Med. Arch.*, **8,** Art. 8.

Helms, J. M. (1987) Acupuncture for the management of primary dysmenorrhea. *Obstet. Gynaecol.*, **69,** 51–56.

Hersh, E. V., Ochs, H., Quinn, P. *et al.* (1993). Narcotic receptor blockade and its effect on the analgesic response to placebo and ibuprofen after oral surgery. *Oral Surg. Oral Med. Oral Pathol. Oral Radiol. Endod.*, **75,** 539–546.

Hesse, J., Mogelvang, B. and Simonsen, H. (1994). Acupuncture versus metoprolol in migraine prophylaxis: a randomised trial of trigger point inactivation. *J. Int. Med.*, **235,** 451–456.

Hester, J. (1998). Acupuncture in the pain clinic. In *Medical Acupuncture. A Western Scientific Approach* (J. Filshie and A. White, eds), pp. 319–340. Edinburgh: Churchill Livingstone.

Hong, C. Z. (1994). Lidocaine injection versus dry needling to myofascial trigger point. The importance of the local twitch response. *Am. J. Phys. Med.*, **73,** 256–263.

Hong, C. Z. and Hsueh, T. C. (1996). Difference in pain relief after trigger point injections in myofascial pain patients with and without fibromyalgia. *Arch. Phys. Med. Rehabil.*, 77, 1161–1166.

Hong, C. Z., Kuan, T. S., Chen, J. T. and Chen, S. M. (1997). Referred pain elicited by palpation and by needling of myofascial trigger points, a comparison. *Arch. Phys. Med. Rehabil.*, **78,** 957–960.

Hubbard, D. R. and Berkoff, G. M. (1993). Myofascial trigger points show EMG activity. *Spine.*, **18,** 1803–1807.

Itoh, M. and Lee, M. H. M. (1971). The epidemiology of disability as related to rehabilitation medicine. In *Krusen's Handbook of Physical Medicine and Rehabilitation* (F. T. Kottke and J. F. Lehmann, eds). Philadelphia: W. B. Saunders.

Jacobsen, S., Bartels, E. M. and Danneskoild-Samsoe, B. (1991). Single cell morphology of muscle in patients with chronic muscle pain. *Scand. J. Rheumatol.*, **20,** 336–343.

Jaeger, B. and Reeves, J. L. (1986). Quantification of changes in myofascial trigger point sensitivity with the pressure algometer following passive stretch. *Pain*, **27,** 203–210.

Jobst, K., Chen, J. H., McPherson, K., Arrowsmith, J. *et al.* (1986). Controlled trial of acupuncture for disabling breathlessness. *Lancet*, **328,** 1416–1419.

Johansson, K., Lindgren, I., Widner, H. *et al.* (1993). Can sensory stimulation improve the functional outcome in stroke patients? *Neurology*, **43,** 2189–2192.

Jones, A. K. P., Brown, W. D., Friston, K. J. *et al.* (1991). Cortical and subcortical localization of response to pain in man using positron emission tomography. *Proc. R. Soc. Lond.*, **244,** 39–44.

Katz, R. L., Kao, C. Y., Spiegel, H. and Katz, G. J. (1974). Pain, acupuncture, hypnosis. In *Advances in Neurology*, vol. 4 . *International Symposium on Pain* (J. J. Bonica, ed.), pp. 819–827. New York: Raven.

Kelleher, C. J., Filshie, J., Burton, G. *et al.* (1994). Acupuncture and the treatment of irritative bladder symptoms. *Acupunct. Med.*, **12,** 9–12.

Kellgren, J. H. (1938). Observations on referred pain arising from muscle. *Clin. Sci.*, **3,** 175–190.

Kelly, M. (1945). The nature of fibrositis, 1. The myalgic lesion and its secondary effects, a reflex theory. *Ann. Rheum. Dis.*, **5,** 1–7.

Klarskov, P. (1987). Enkephalin inhibits presynaptically the contractility of urinary tract smooth muscle. *Br. J. Urol.*,**59,** 31–35.

Kleijnen, J., Ter Riet, G. and Knipschild, P. (1991). Acupuncture and asthma. A review of controlled trials. *Thorax*, **46,** 799–802.

Knottnerus, J. A. and Dinant, G. J. (1997). Medicine based evidence, a prerequisite for evidence based medicine. *Br. Med. J.*, **315**, 1109–1110.

Koizumi, K. and McC Brooks, C. (1984). The spinal cord and the autonomic nervous system. In *Handbook of the Spinal Cord*, vols 2 and 3 (Davidoff, R. A. ed.), pp. 779–795. New York: Marcel Dekker.

Kruse, R. A. Jr and Christiansen, J. A. (1992). Thermographic imaging of myofascial trigger points, a follow-up study. *Arch. Phys. Med. Rehabil.*, **73**, 819–823.

Lange, F. and Eversbusch, G. (1921). Die bedeutung der Muskelhärten für die allgemeine Praxis. *Müench. Med. Wochenschr.*, **68,** 418–420.

Lao, L., Bergman, S., Langenberg, P. *et al.* (1995) Efficacy of Chinese acupuncture on postoperative oral surgery pain. *Oral Surg. Oral Med. Oral Pathol. Oral Radiol. Endodont.*, **79,** 423–428.

Lazarou, J., Pomeranz, B. H. and Corey, P. N. (1998). Incidence of adverse drug reactions in hospitalised patients. A meta analysis of prospective studies. *JAMA*, **279,** 1200–1205.

Lee, Y. H., Lee W. C., Chen, M. T. *et al.* (1992). Acupuncture in the treatment of renal colic. *J. Urol.*, **14,** 6–18.

Levine, J. D., Gormley, J. and Fields, H. L. (1976). Observations on the analgesic effects of needle puncture (acupuncture). *Pain*, **2,** 149–159.

Levine, J. D., Gordon, N. C., Bornstein, J. C. and Fields, H. L. (1979). Role of pain in placebo analgesia. *Proc. Natl. Acad. Sci. USA*, **76,** 3528–3531.

Lewit, K. and Simons, D. G. (1984). Myofascial pain, relief by post-isometric relaxation. *Arch. Phys. Med. Rehabil.*, **65,** 452–456.

Lewith, G. T. and Vincent, C. (1996). On the evaluation of the clinical effects of acupuncture, a problem reassessed and a framework for future research. *J. Altern. Comp. Med.*, **2,** 79–100.

Lewith, G. T. and Vincent, C. A. (1998). The clinical evaluation of acupuncture. In *Medical Acupuncture. A Western Scientific Approach* (J. Filshie and A. White, eds), pp. 205–224. Edinburgh: Churchill Livingstone.

Ligouri, R., Krarup, C. and Trojaborg, W. (1992). Determination of the segmental sensory and motor innervation of the lumbosacral spinal nerves. An electrophysiological study. *Brain*, **115,** 915–934.

List, T. and Helkimo, M. (1987). Acupuncture in the treatment of patients with chronic facial pain and mandibular dysfunction. *Swed. Dent. J.*, **11,** 83–92.

List, T. and Helkimo, M. (1992). Acupuncture and occlusal splint therapy in the treatment of craniomandibular disorders. II. A 1-year follow-up study. *Acta Odontol. Scand.*, **50,** 375–385.

List, T., Helkimo, M. and Karlsson, R. (1993). Pressure pain thresholds in patients with craniomandibular disorders before and after treatment with acupuncture and occlusal splint therapy, a controlled clinical study. *J. Orofac. Pain*,**7,** 275–282.

McCain, G. A. (1993). Chronic musculoskeletal pain syndromes – overlapping features of myofascial pain and fibromyalgia. Abstract – 7th World Congress on Pain, p. 495.

MacDonald, A. J., Macrae, K. D., Master, B. R. and Rubin, A. P. (1983). Superficial acupuncture in the relief of chronic low back pain. *Ann. R. Coll. Surg. Engl.*, **65,** 44–46.

McMillan, C. M. (1998). Acupuncture for nausea and vomiting. In *Medical Acupuncture. A Western Scientific Approach* (J. Filshie and A. White, eds), pp. 295–317. Edinburgh: Churchill Livingstone.

McNulty, W. H., Gervirtz, R. N., Hubbard, D. R. and Berkoff, G. M. (1994). Needle electromyographic evaluation of trigger point response to a psychological stressor. *Psychophysiology*, **31,** 313–316.

Madell, J. R. (1975). Acupuncture for sensorineural hearing loss. *Arch. Otolaryngol.*, **101,** 441–445.

Magni, G., Calderion, C., Rigatti-Luchini, S. and Merskey, H. (1990). Chronic musculoskeletal pain and depressive symptoms in the general population. An analysis of the 1st National Health and Nutrition Examination Survey data. *Pain*, **43**, 299–307.

Mann, F. (1992). *Reinventing Acupuncture. A New Concept of Ancient Medicine.* Oxford: Butterworth Heinemann.

Melzack, R. and Wall, P. D. (1965). Pain mechanisms, a new theory. *Science*, **150**, 971–979.

Melzack, R., Stillwell, D. M. and Fox, E. J. (1977). Trigger points and acupuncture points for pain, correlations and implications. *Pain*, **3**, 3–23.

Molsberger, A. and Hille, E. (1994). The analgesic effect of acupuncture in chronic tennis elbow pain. *Br. J. Rheumatol.*, **33**, 1162–1165.

Moore, M. E. and Berk, S. N. (1976). Acupuncture for chronic shoulder pain. An experimental study with attention to the role of placebo and hypnotic susceptibility. *Ann. Int. Med.*, **84**, 381–384.

Murray, K. H. A. (1983). Effect of naloxone induced opioid blockade on idiopathic detrusor instability. *Urology*, **22**, 329–331.

Murray, K. H. A. and Feneley, R. C. A. (1982). Endorphins. A role in lower urinary tract function? The effect of opioid blockade on the detrusor and urethral sphincter mechanisms. *Br. J. Urol.*, **54**, 638–640.

Nice, D. A., Riddle, D. L., Lamb, R. L. *et al.* (1993). Intertester reliability of judgements of the presence of trigger points in patients with low back pain. *Arch. Phys. Med. Rehabil.*, **73**, 893–898.

Njoo, K. H. and Van der Does, D. (1995). The occurrence of inter-rater reliability of myofascial trigger points in the quadratus lumborum and gluteus medius, a prospective study in non-specific low back pain patients and controls in general practice. *Pain*, **58**, 317–323.

Nogier, P. F. M. (1972). *Treatise of Auriculotherapy*. Moulin-le-Metz, France: Maisonneuve.

Oleson, T. D., Kroening R. J. and Bresler, D. E. (1980). An experimental evaluation of auricular diagnosis. The somatotopic mapping of musculoskeletal pain at ear acupuncture points. *Pain*, **8**, 217–229.

Patel, M., Gutzwiller, F., Paccaud, F. and Marazzi, A. (1989). A meta-analysis of acupuncture for chronic pain. *Int. J. Epidemiol.*, **18**, 900–906.

Petrie, J. P. and Langley, G. B. (1983). Acupuncture in the treatment of chronic cervical pain, a pilot study. *Clin. Exp. Rheumatol.*, **1**, 333–336.

Phillips II, L. H. and Park, T. S. (1991). Electrophysiologic mapping of the segmental anatomy of the muscles of the lower extremity. *Muscle Nerve*, **14**, 1213–1218.

Phillips II, L. H. and Park, T. S. (1993). Electrophysiological mapping of the segmental innervation of the saphenous and sural nerves. *Muscle Nerve*, **16**, 827–831.

Picalov, A. A. and Kharin, V. V. (1994). Use of spinal manipulative therapy in the treatment of duodenal ulcer, a pilot study. *J. Manipulative Physiol. Ther.*, **17**, 310–313.

Price, D. D., Rafii, A., Watkins, L. R. and Buckingham, B. (1984). A psychophysical analysis of acupuncture analgesia. *Pain*, **19**, 27–42.

Qiu, M. L., Sheng, C. R. and Li, N. (1979). Researches on treatment of acute bacillary dysentery by acupuncture. *Abstracts of 1st National Symposium of Acupuncture, Beijing*, pp. 2–5.

Reeves, J. L., Jaeger, B. and Graff-Radford, S. B. (1986). Reliability of the pressure algometer as a measure of myofascial trigger point sensitivity. *Pain*, **24**, 313–321.

Richardson, P. H. (1990). Pain and the placebo effect. *Frontiers of Pain*, **II**, 1–2.

Roberts, A. H. D. G., Kewman, D. G., Mercier, L. and Hovell, M. (1993). The power of non-specific effects in healing, implications for psychosocial and biological treatments. *Clin. Psychol. Rev.*, **13**, 375–391.

Roppolo, J. R., Booth, A. M. and De Groot, W. C. (1983). The effects of naloxone on the neural control of the urinary bladder of the cat. *Brain Res.*, **264**, 355–358.

Sackett, D. (1979) Bias in analytical research. *J. Chron. Dis.*, **32**, 51–63.

Sato, A. and Schmidt, R. F. (1973). Somatosympathetic reflexes, afferent fibres, central pathways, discharge characteristics. *Physiol. Rev.*, **53**, 916–943.

Sato, A., Sato, Y. and Susuki, A. (1992). Mechanisms of the reflex inhibition of micturition contractions of the urinary bladder elicited by acupuncture-like stimulation in anesthetised rats. *Neurosci. Res.*, **15,** 189–198.

Schade, H. (1921). Untersuchungen in der Erkältungstrage, III. Uber den Rheumatismus, insbesondereden Muskelrheumatismus (Myogelosis). *Müench. Med. Wochenschr.*, **68,** 95–99.

Sola, A. E., Rodenberger, M. L. and Gettys, B. B. (1955). Incidence of hypersensitive areas in posterior shoulder muscles. *Am. J. Phys. Med.*, **3,** 585–590.

Taub, H. A. (1975). Acupuncture and sensorineural hearing loss, a review. *J. Speech Hear. Dis.*, **40**, 427–433.

Ter Riet, G., Kleijnen, J. and Knipschild, P. (1990a). Acupuncture and chronic pain. A criteria based meta-analysis. *J. Clin. Epidemiol.*, **43,** 1191–1199.

Ter Riet, G., Kleijnen, J. and Knipschild, P. (1990b). A meta-analysis of studies into the effect of acupuncture on addiction. *Br. J. Gen. Pract.*, **40**, 379–382.

Ter Riet, G., de Craen, A. J. M., dee Boer, A. and Kessels, A. G. H. (1998). Is placebo analgesia mediated by endogenous opioids? A systematic review. *Pain*, **76,** 273–275.

Thomas, M., (1995). Treatment of Pain with Acupuncture, Factors Influencing Outcome. PhD Thesis, Karolinska Institutet, Stockholm.

Thomas, M. (1997). Acupuncture studies on pain. *Acupunct. Med.*, **15,** 23–31.

Thomas, M. and Lundeberg, T. (1994). Importance of modes of acupuncture in the treatment of chronic nociceptive low back pain. *Acta Anaesthesiol. Scand.*, **38**, 63–69.

Thomas, M., Eriksson, S. V. and Lundeberg, T. (1991). A comparative study of diazepam and acupuncture in patients with osteoarthritis pain, a placebo controlled study. *Am. J. Chin. Med.*, **19,** 95–100.

Thomas, M., Lundeberg, T., Bjork, G. and Lundstrom-Lindstedt, V. (1995). Pain and discomfort in primary dysmenorrhea is reduced by pre-emptive acupuncture or low frequency TENS. *Eur. J. Phys. Med. Rehabil.*, **5,** 71–76.

Thompson, J. W. and Filshie, J. (1997). Transcutaneous electrical nerve stimulation (TENS) and acupuncture. In *Oxford Textbook of Palliative Medicine* (D. Doyle, G. Hanks and N. MacDonald, eds), pp. 421–437. Oxford: Oxford University Press.

Tougas, G., Yuan, L. Y., Radamaker, J. W. *et al.* (1992). Effect of acupuncture on gastric acid secretion in healthy male volunteers. *Dig. Dis. Sci.*, **37,** 1576–1582.

Travell, J. (1976). Myofascial trigger points, clinical view. In *Advances in Pain Research and Therapy*, vol. 1 (J. J. Bonica and D Albe-Fessard, eds), pp. 919–926. New York: Raven.

Travell, J. G. and Simons, D. G. (1983). *Myofascial Pain and Dysfunction. The Trigger Point Manual.* Baltimore: Williams and Wilkins.

Tschopp, W. P. and Gysin, C. (1996). Local injection therapy in 107 patients with myofascial pain syndrome of the head and neck. *J. Oto-Rhino-Laryngol. Rel. Spec.*, **58,** 306–310.

Tunks, E., McCain, G. A., Hart, L. E. *et al.* (1995). The reliability of examination for tenderness in patients with myofascial pain, chronic fibromyalgia and controls. *J. Rheumatol.*, **22,** 944–952.

Urwin, M., Symmons, D. P. M., Allison, T. *et al.* (1998) Estimating the burden of musculoskeletal disorders in the community, the comparative prevalence of symptoms at different anatomical sites and the relationship to social deprivation. *Ann. Rheum. Dis.* **57** (11), 649–655.

Vickers, A. J. (1996). Can acupuncture have specific effects on health? A systematic review of acupuncture antiemesis trials. *J. R. Soc. Med.*, **89,** 303–311.

Vincent, C. A. (1989). A controlled trial of the treatment of migraine by acupuncture. *Clin. J. Pain.*, **5,** 305–312.

Vincent, C. (1990). Credibility assessments in trials of acupuncture. *Comp. Med. Res.*, **4,** 8–11.

Vincent C. A. (1992). Acupuncture research, Why do it? *Comp. Med. Res.*, **6,** 21–24.

Vincent, C. A. and Lewith, G. T. (1995). Placebo controls for acupuncture studies. *J. R. Soc. Med.*, **88,** 199–202.

Virchow, R. (1852) Ueber parenchymatösa Entzündung. *Arch. Path. Anat.*, **4,** 261–279.

Wall, P. D. (1994). The placebo and the placebo response. In *Textbook of Pain*, 3rd edn. (P. D. Wall and R. Melzack, eds), pp. 1297–1308. New York: Churchill Livingstone.

Ward, A. (1996). Spontaneous electrical activity at combined acupuncture and myofascial trigger point sites. *Acupunct. Med*, **14,** 75–79.

White, A. R. and Ernst, E. (1998) A trial method for assessing the adequacy of acupuncture treatments. *Alt. Ther. Health Med*, **4,** 66–71.

White, A. R., Eddleston, C., Hardie, R. *et al.* (1996). A pilot study of acupuncture for tension headache, using a novel placebo. *Acupunct. Med.*, **14,** 11–15.

Williamson, L., Yudkin, P., Livingstone, R. *et al.* (1996). Hayfever treatment in general practice – randomised controlled trial comparing standardised Western acupuncture with sham acupuncture. *Acupunct. Med.*, **14,** 6–10.

Wolfe, F., Simons, D. G., Fricton, J. *et al.* (1992). The fibromyalgia and myofascial pain syndromes, a preliminary study of tender points and trigger points in persons with fibromyalgia, myofascial pain syndrome and no disease. *J. Rheumatol.*, **19,** 944–951.

Wreje, U. and Brorsson, B. (1995). A multicenter randomised controlled trial of injections of sterile water and saline for chronic myofascial pain syndromes. *Pain*, **61,** 441–444.

Wyon, Y., Lindgren, R., Lundeberg, T., Hammar, M. (1995). Effects of acupuncture on climacteric vasomotor symptoms, quality of life and urinary-excretion of neuropeptides among postmenopausal women. *Menopause Journal of the North American Menopause Society*, **2**(1), 3–12.

Yamamoto, Y, (1989). New scalp acupuncture. *Acupunct. Med.*, **6,** 46–48.

Yamamoto, T., Yamamoto, H. (1998). *Yamamoto New Scalp Acupuncture YNSA*. Axel Springer Japan Publishing Inc.

Yao, T. (1993). Acupuncture and somatic nerve stimulation, mechanism underlying effects on cardiovascular and renal activities. *Scand. J. Rehabil. Med.*, **29,** 7–18.

Yarnell, S. K., Waylonis, G. W. and Rink, T. L. (1976). Acupuncture effect on neurosensory deafness. *Arch. Phys. Med. Rehabil.*, **57,** 166–168.

Zhang, T. Q., Jin, A. D. and Li, S. Se. (1979). The curative effects of acupuncture on bacillary dysentery in Rhesus monkey and the experimental study of its mechanisms. *Abstracts of 1st National Symposium of Acupuncture. Beijing*, pp. 40–41.

3

Neurophysiology of acupuncture analgesia

Adrian White

Introduction

It is important to explore the neurophysiology of acupuncture for several reasons. First, it can provide the basis for choosing the most effective treatment methods for different conditions; second, it may explain phenomena that may be observed during treatment; third, it suggests hypotheses for more experimental studies to improve therapy still further; and fourth, acupuncture is likely to only gain respectability in a scientific context if it can be convincingly explained by neurophysiological mechanisms. However, it must be accepted that even the most precise mechanism of acupuncture still does not provide evidence for the clinical effectiveness: this requires evidence from clinical studies.

Three independent discoveries during the decade following 1965 by chance together put acupuncture 'on the map'. The Gate Control Theory provided a possible framework (Melzack and Wall, 1965), the opioid peptides provided a possible mechanism (Hughes *et al.*, 1975), and surgical analgesia provided a possible model (Dimond, 1971).

Neurophysiological research: is it 'acupuncture'?

The western world was astonished by television documentaries of operations being performed on fully conscious patients in China with apparently only acupuncture for anaesthetic. Laboratory animal models of acupuncture analgesia were soon developed (Peking Acupuncture Anaesthesia Co-ordinating Group, 1973) and have permitted a vast number of elegant experiments to explore the analgesia that results from electrical nerve stimulation. The analgesia model was derived from clinical experience with acupuncture; acupuncture needles acted as a convenient electrode for these experiments; therefore much of this neurophysiological research was regarded as research into acupuncture. There are, however, several differences between nerve stimulation as performed in laboratories and as performed in clinical acupuncture:

- Anatomy and physiology of nociceptive mechanisms differ somewhat between species. For example, rats and other lower animals can be rendered analgesic by sheer fright, or by electric shocks on the feet.

- There is no way to tell if animals experience needle sensation, yet this sensation may be critical for clinical acupuncture.
- Standard 'human' needles of 0.3 mm diameter are likely to be considerably more traumatic to the rat's tibialis anterior, which is only 5 mm thick, than that of the human, which is at least 50 mm thick (although the relative size of needle and individual muscle fibre would be the same for both species).
- The sensation of pain in humans depends on the interaction of a variety of psychological and physical factors. Examining isolated tracts, nuclei or cells in animal preparations gives only a small part of the picture.
- Experimental pain has many differences from clinical pain, because nociceptive mechanisms undergo profound and rapid changes once a pathological process begins.

Despite the shortcomings of the model using experimental analgesia, it does provide the first step to exploring the mechanisms of pain relief. It is reassuring that the model has proved useful in other contexts, for example in assessing novel analgesic drugs (Gracely, 1991), but we should remain cautious in relating laboratory findings to clinical practice.

Terminology

In laboratory experiments, nerves are frequently stimulated by electrical current, applied either through pads or needles, to the intact skin or to a nerve that has been exposed by dissection. There is an argument for restricting the term 'acupuncture' to clinical practice alone, to distinguish it from other methods and terms, such as sensory stimulation, dry needling, peripheral nerve stimulation, electrostimulation, etc. While this may be logical and strictly speaking correct, it has not been possible to find a single, unequivocal term that would be universally acceptable. Therefore the terms 'acupuncture' and 'acupuncture analgesia' will be used in this chapter to describe all forms of stimulation in clinical and laboratory circumstances, with the following exception.

Transcutaneous electrical nerve stimulation (TENS) overlaps substantially electroacupuncture (EA), the former being applied through carbon rubber pad electrodes rather than needles and (conventionally) using higher frequency stimulation. It is generally agreed that the clinical effect of TENS is usually substantially different from that of acupuncture: TENS produces a rapid onset of analgesia with no sustained effect; the analgesia does not accumulate over repeated treatments; the analgesia is generally not reversible with naloxone. Ishimaru *et al.* (1995) found that the degree of analgesia produced by electrical stimulation through TENS pads was considerably smaller than the equivalent stimulus given through deep needles. This chapter has been written on the assumption that TENS and EA have different clinical effects, and will concentrate on the latter. Readers who wish to find out more specifically about TENS will find an excellent summary of the application and neurophysiology of TENS given by Woolf and Thompson (1994).

Acupuncture as stimulus

The strength of the stimulation applied with acupuncture needles varies considerably among different practitioners. At its mildest, one needle is gently placed in subcutaneous tissues and left for less than a minute (Baldry, 1993). More typically, half a dozen or more needles are placed in deeper tissues, usually muscle, gently stimulated until needle sensation is elicited, and then left for up to 20 minutes. At its strongest, the needle is thrust down to bone and agitated, 'pecking' the periosteum in a painful way. In addition, electrical stimulation may be used, sometimes at a level that is just detectable to the patient, sometimes strong enough to produce muscle contractions, and sometimes just below the threshold of pain.

Acupuncture points

Acupuncture points are not shown as precise anatomical locations in earliest Chinese texts; this only happened later (Mann, 1992). Currently, acupuncture students are taught 361 precise locations where tradition states that needles should be placed for optimal effect. Local anaesthetic abolishes that effect (Chiang *et al.*, 1973). These locations might therefore be expected to show some uniform receptor organ, consistent arrangement of nerve fibres or correspondence with other neuromuscular phenomena.

In order to examine this correlation, Liu *et al.* (1975) compared 31 selected acupuncture points with motor points (defined as locations where the muscle could be stimulated with smallest electrical current). Acupuncturists and neurophysiologists independently identified the points on a volunteer and marked them with invisible ink. After revealing the ink with UV light, the position of the marks was compared: ten of the points were within 4 mm of each other, six were within 10 mm but the remaining 15 were more than 10 mm apart. Clearly, acupuncture points are by no means the same as motor points.

Another attempt at explaining points was made by an anatomist, Dung (1984). He produced a list of ten nerve conformations that could be identified at acupuncture points: however, this was not a systematic examination of all acupuncture points, no data such as frequency was presented, and there was no attempt to explain how the different nerve conformations might correlate with the use of points in practice. As mentioned in Chapter 2, Melzack *et al.* (1977) found that acupuncture points correlated with trigger points in 100% of cases, allowing for a 3-cm discrepancy. However, there are inconsistencies: for example, the three known trigger points in the infraspinatus (Travell and Simons, 1983) do not all lie within 3 cm of the local acupuncture point, SI 11.

Chan (1984) conducted a cautious, objective review of the literature and found insufficient evidence to conclude that acupuncture points have consistent anatomical features.

Acupuncture points and skin resistance

Acupuncture points are located in practice either by their anatomical location or by tenderness. Some workers have suggested that they can be identified by changes in skin resistance. On the one hand, it is easy to find small circumscribed areas of skin which have a low electrical resistance. Chan (1984) stated that these areas of low resistance were believed by Chinese researchers to represent traditional acupuncture points. These observations were elaborated into a novel system of therapy in Japan called Ryodoraku, in which disease of visceral organs is said to be reflected by abnormal electrical resistance at corresponding points of the skin.

However, Chan (1984) points out that measurements of skin resistance can be confounded by many factors such as the cross-sectional area of the electrode, the amount of pressure and the contact time. The stratum corneum layer of the epidermis contributes over 90% of skin resistance and its structure is readily distorted by pressure applied during measurement. Subsequently, the skin resistance of acupuncture points was carefully and systematically explored by Cho and Chun (1994). Potential errors caused by condition of skin, pressure of electrode, diurnal variation, etc. were minimized. Repeated measurements of skin resistance at eight traditional acupuncture points in ten healthy volunteers produced inconsistent and unreliable results: no significant patterns or correlations were found, either for opposite sides of individuals, or between different individuals.

Acupuncture meridians

There have been a number of attempts to validate the concept of meridians by demonstrating measurable changes in one form or another. Darras *et al.* (1993) concluded that meridian pathways could be marked by injecting radioactively labelled technetium into acupuncture points, and that these pathways were separate from lymph vessels. Wu *et al.* (1994) found that technetium uptake was faster from certain acupuncture points than from non-points, but that its movement thereafter was explained entirely by the venous system. Cohen *et al.* (1995) found that the electrical resistance along one meridian in the arm was less than that between non-acupuncture points. Overall, such exploratory studies have not as yet provided any consistent evidence for the existence of meridians.

Needle sensation

Many practitioners consider that, for acupuncture to be most effective, the needles should elicit needle sensation. Needle sensation is an unusual and somewhat unpleasant sensation, ranging from numbness to distension and aching, and finally soreness or pain. It may occur when a needle is inserted without stimulation (Takeda and Wessel, 1994), but is usually induced by manipulating the needle in a rotational direction or by lifting and thrusting. It is possible to elicit needle sensation by inserting needles into areas that are not recognized as acupuncture points (Vincent *et al.*, 1989). At the same time that needle sensation is felt by the patient, the acupuncturist can usually detect that the needle is being gripped by muscle tissues. However, needle sensation does not seem to depend on muscle contraction, because Chan (1984) reported that patients with musculodystrophy could feel needle sensation even though muscle contraction did not occur, as confirmed by electromyography.

What nerve is stimulated?

Most practising acupuncturists would say that their patients might feel discomfort from the needles, but not pain: this makes A delta fibres the most likely candidate (Bowsher, 1987). There is general support for the notion that acupuncture stimulates A delta fibres, either from free nerve endings in the skin (Baldry, 1993) or from high-threshold ergoreceptors in muscle (Andersson and Lundeberg, 1995). Wang *et al.* (1985) recorded action potentials in the median nerve produced by acupuncture in the forearm, and correlated these with the sensations described by the subjects. The action potentials were categorized into different nerve fibre types. The conclusions were that numbness was conveyed by A gamma fibres, distension and heaviness by A delta fibres and soreness by C fibres (Table 3.1).

It is interesting to note that, after needling, discharges generally lasted only a few minutes. Occasionally the discharge would last for 10 minutes, particularly after needling deeper points.

Chung *et al.* (1984) studied which fibre type needs to be stimulated to produce analgesia. Peripheral nerves in the legs of monkeys were stimulated with stepwise increases in intensity, while potentials were recorded in the afferent nerve. The effect of each intensity was measured by the inhibition of the response of spinothalamic tract cells to noxious stimulus. Stimulation of A alpha and A beta fibres produced a small but significant inhibition; A delta fibre stimulation produced a greatly enhanced inhibition that outlasted the stimulation; and finally, increasing the stimulation intensity to include C fibres produced another small

Table 3.1 Correlation between fibre type, physiological function, and role in acupuncture analgesia and needle sensation (after J. Thompson, personal communication)

Nerve type	*Function*	*Evidence for role in acupuncture analgesia*	*Needle sensation experienced (Wang* et al., *1985)*
A alpha	muscle spindle	Lu, 1983	
A beta	touch, vibration	Lu, 1983; Toda and Ichioka, 1978	
A gamma	flower spray, muscle spindle		numbness
A delta	pinprick, cold; pressure; muscle ergoreceptor	Chung *et al.*, 1984; Baldry, 1993; Bowsher, 1987; Andersson and Lundeberg, 1995	distension, heaviness
C	deep pain, itch	Liu *et al.*, 1986	soreness

increase in inhibition. This suggests that acupuncture analgesia depends principally on A delta fibre stimulation.

On the other hand, other evidence suggests that other fibres may be important. Toda and Ichioka (1978) measured the analgesic effect of 45-Hz electrical stimulation to the Hoku point in the cat paw: analgesia was measured as the jaw-opening response to a noxious stimulus. Nerve conduction times in the brachial nerve were used to identify which afferent fibres were involved at different intensities of stimulation. Maximum analgesia was achieved by stimulating A beta fibres; increasing the stimulus to include A delta fibres did not increase the analgesia further. In a somewhat similar experiment with cats and rabbits, Lu (1983) inserted needles into ST 36 and adjusted their position precisely until they produced analgesia. From the velocity of the impulses in the peroneal nerve, it was concluded that manual acupuncture stimulated A alpha and beta, but not A delta, nerve fibres. Evidence for the importance of C fibre stimulation was provided by Liu *et al.* (1992), who found that stimulation had to be strong enough to stimulate C fibres before the brainstem cells were activated leading to descending inhibition (see below).

Kawakita and Gotoh (1996) presented evidence suggesting that the polymodal receptor is responsible for the flare surrounding the acupuncture needle and for the needle sensation. They suggested that the acupuncture effect depends on stimulating polymodal receptors rather than any particular nerve fibre. This would provide a rational basis for the use of stimulation by heat (moxibustion).

In summary, there is an assumption that the nerves most closely involved in the acupuncture response are the A delta fibres, but this has not been proved beyond doubt.

Pain mechanisms and nociceptive control

Background

The evolutionary 'purpose' of pain is to warn of physical injury and to stimulate evasive action. Throughout the first two-thirds of the twentieth century, pain mechanisms were explained by the **specificity theory**: pain was regarded as the automatic outcome from activation of pain **receptors** stimulating pain **pathways** to a pain **centre** in the brain. However, as Melzack and Wall (1973) argued powerfully, this theory is contradicted both by everyday experience and by clinical observation. On the one hand, injury often occurs without causing pain, for example on the sports field or more dramatically in battle, where traumatic limb amputation has occurred completely painlessly. On the other hand, chronic pain can and frequently does persist long after the original inflammation or injury has healed.

The specificity theory has been replaced by the Gate Control Theory of pain (Melzack and Wall, 1965). A stimulus is not regarded as essentially 'painful'. Rather, it indicates trauma and is therefore termed 'nociceptive'. Individual nociceptor nerve fibres may respond to a single stimulus such as strong mechanical pressure or to heat or cold, or they may be polymodal, i.e. respond to many stimuli. Nociceptive fibres generally project onto spinal neurones, which may respond to a variety of stimuli – they have a wide dynamic range. The nociceptive stimulus is processed or 'modulated' on its passage through the CNS and may or may not result in the unpleasant experience that we recognize as pain. Modulation is the result of the balance of various inhibitory and facilitatory mechanisms throughout the CNS. The level of pain experienced may be influenced by simultaneous activity elsewhere in the CNS, or from psychological factors including previous experience of pain, conditioning, expectation, fear, desire, as well as cultural and genetic influences. The process of preventing noxious stimuli from reaching consciousness is referred to as 'nociceptive control'. There is now considerably greater understanding of the mechanisms by which peripheral stimulation can exert nociceptive control. By contrast, the understanding of chronic pain and of the mechanisms of psychological influences on pain is still relatively limited.

Nociceptive stimuli activate small nerve fibres, including the unmyelinated C fibres and the myelinated A delta fibres. Stimulation of the primitive C fibres produces pain with a profound quality ('slow, deep or chronic pain') and a strong emotional effect. It may be inhibited by the action of larger myelinated fibres, including the A delta and the A beta groups. These developed much later (in evolutionary terms) than C fibres. There follows a description of the nociceptive pathways, with particular reference to the role of acupuncture.

C fibres

Small, unmyelinated C fibres are the most numerous fibres in mammalian afferent nerves. They convey impulses from free nerve endings, which are widely distributed under the skin and in deep tissues including the viscera. These free nerve endings are either high-threshold pressure receptors or polymodal nociceptors that respond to heavy pressure, heat or chemicals. Their threshold may be reduced in certain disease states, a process known as 'sensitization'. Sensitization appears to be stimulated by nerve growth factor which is released during inflammation: nerves respond to light pressure which was previously subthreshold ('allodynia').

When C fibres reach the spinal cord, they send branches a few segments in both rostral and caudal directions, giving off twigs. The twigs terminate in the dorsal horn, making synaptic contact with the substantia gelatinosa (SG) cells in lamina II (Figure 3.1).

C fibres release the amino acids glutamate and aspartate as transmitters. The response of the SG cells varies according to the balance of inhibitory or excitatory neuromodulators present on the cell membrane at that moment, acting via their opposing ability to influence ion channels. Changes in the ion channel properties may either produce a change in the resting membrane potential (thus altering the threshold of depolarization) or alter the activity of membrane receptors.

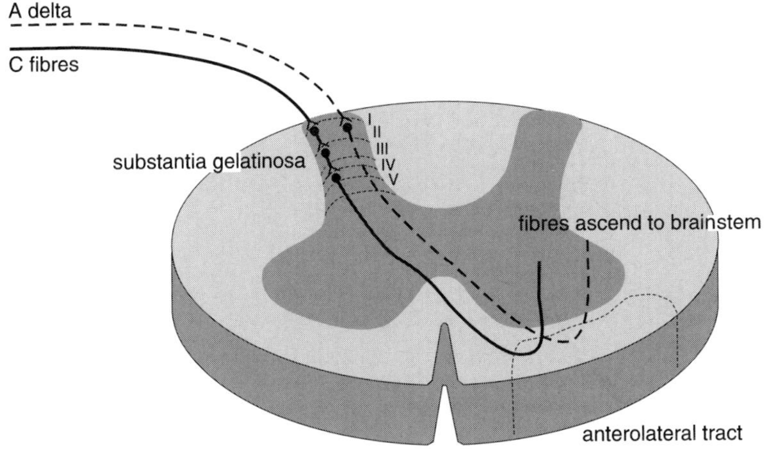

Figure 3.1 Diagram of segment of spinal cord showing connections and routes of C and A delta fibres.

SG cells possess several classes of receptor for glutamate and aspartate. The activity of two receptors is understood in some detail, and underlies the difference between acute and chronic pain, at least in part. In **acute** pain, glutamate released by nociceptive impulses stimulates the α-amino-3-hydroxy-5-methyl-4-isoxalone propionic acid (AMPA) receptor (Figure 3.2).

The AMPA receptor responds to impulses on a strictly one-to-one basis. In **chronic** pain, repeated C fibre stimulation leads to the release not only of the amino acids but also the peptides substance P, calcitonin gene-related peptide (CGRP) and neurokinin A (Dickenson, 1995). These rapidly activate a second receptor, known as *N*-methyl-d-aspartate

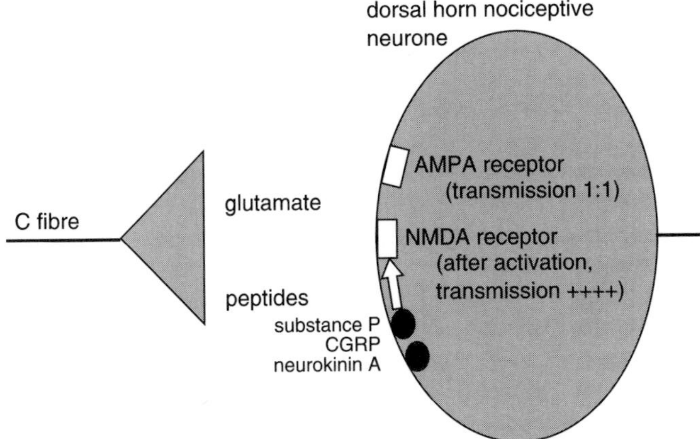

Figure 3.2 Diagram of synapse in substantia gelatinosa, illustrating some transmitters and receptors: peptides activate the NMDA receptor which amplifies the response to incoming nociceptive stimuli. (After Dickenson, 1996, with kind permission of the publishers.)

(NMDA). The NMDA receptor does not respond on a one-to-one basis but produces a greatly amplified signal. In laboratory conditions the amplification can augment responses by 20-fold in magnitude and duration. This is the physiological basis of the phenomenon known as 'central hypersensitivity' in which continuing noxious stimuli cause an exaggerated response.

After being processed in the SG, the nociceptive signal activates the large 'transmission' cells in lamina V. Transmission cells are fewer in number than the fibres in the dorsal root, so sensory information 'converges'. This convergence occurs throughout the afferent system and offers important opportunities for influence, summation and control of nociception.

Transmission cells send their axons to the reticular formation (RF) via the anterolateral tracts on the opposite side of the spinal cord (Figure 3.3).

These tracts are interrupted on their progress by multiple synapses. Reticular cells have large receptive fields and are somatotopically organized in a general way (Soper and Melzack, 1982). The RF is the site of 'arousal' which is an essential precondition for cerebral activity. It is involved in nociception and may play a major role in integrating the experience of pain and the behavioural response.

Nociceptive information then passes forwards, mainly to the intralaminar nuclei of the thalamus, which project diffusely throughout

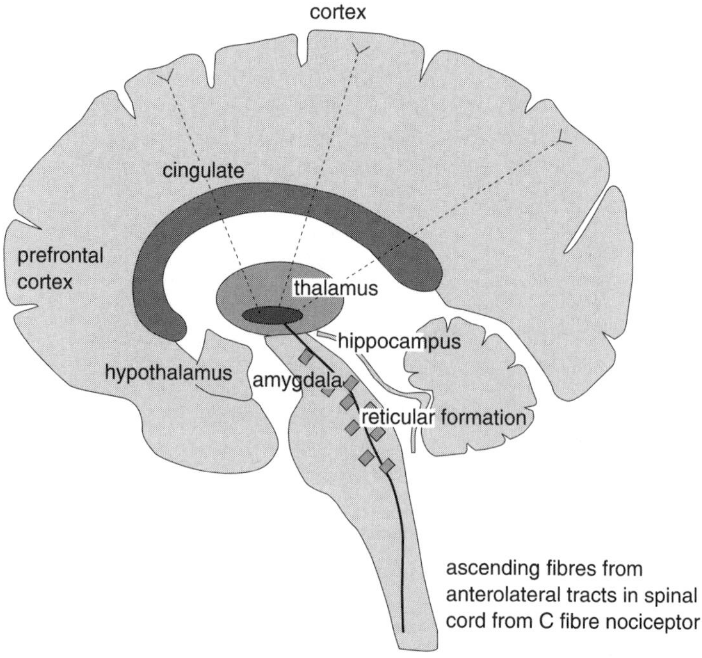

Figure 3.3 Diagram of sagittal section of the brain showing central connections of C fibre nociceptive afferents to: (1) reticular formation; (2) cortex diffusely; (3) limbic system, including thalamus, amygdala, hippocampus, cingulate and prefrontal cortex.

the cerebral cortex. Other fibres pass to the limbic system, including the cingulate gyrus which is the seat of the emotional component of pain (Jones *et al.*, 1991). Thus, noxious stimulation conveyed by the C fibre system leads to a perception of pain that is poorly localized but has considerable emotional impact.

A delta fibres

A delta fibres are activated by pin prick and heavy pressure, heat and cold in skin, and also by high-threshold ergoreceptors in muscle. Some A delta fibres terminate on large cells in lamina I/II in the dorsal horn, others terminate on the transmission cells in lamina V. These cells send their axons (tract fibres) across the cord, over the course of several segments, to join the anterolateral tract near the ventral surface on the opposite side; new fibres are added to the tract on its inner surface, thus maintaining somatotopic representation. A few neurones in the dorsal horn send their axons by different routes, one of which is the propriospinal pathway. Axons in this pathway terminate within the spinal cord, and may prove to have an important role in nociceptive control.

The majority of tract fibres run to the thalamus (ventrobasal nuclei) from where third-order neurones project somatotopically to the primary sensory cortex (Figure 3.4).

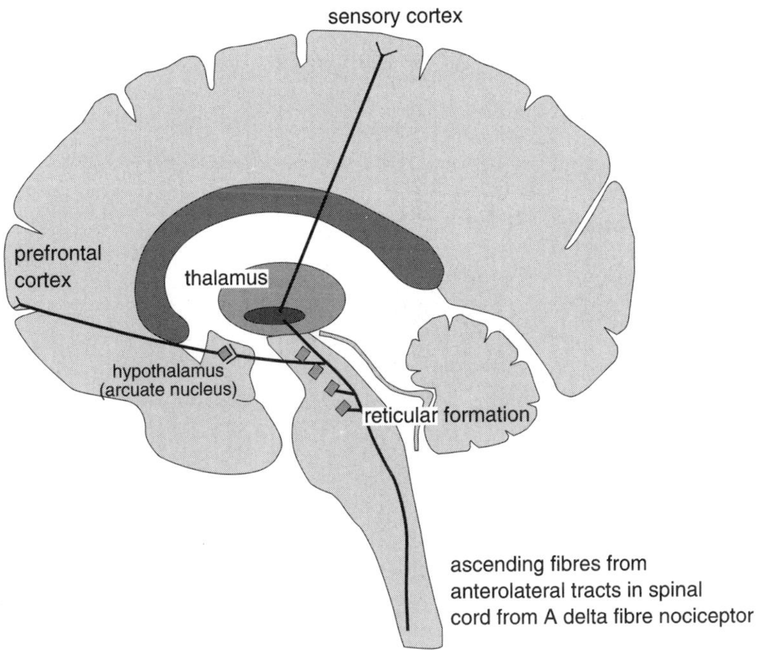

Figure 3.4 Diagram of sagittal section of the brain showing central connections of A delta fibre nociceptor afferents via thalamus to primary sensory cortex, with collaterals to reticular formation, hypothalamus (arcuate nucleus) and prefrontal cortex.

This system provides rapid, accurately localized perception of noxious stimulation without producing much emotional response. However, a substantial minority of fibres terminate on the rostral reticular formation and thence to the thalamus (medial and intralaminar group of nuclei). From here they pass forward to the arcuate nucleus of the hypothalamus and to the prefrontal cortex. This is the upper limit of the afferent arm; it also constitutes the start of the descending inhibitory arm (Takashige *et al.*, 1992, 1993).

A beta fibres

Large A beta fibres have an important function in the body's control of nociceptive input, but, in terms of acupuncture, they are probably only involved in high-frequency electroacupuncture. These fibres are activated by low-threshold stimuli: light touch, joint position sense and vibration. A beta fibres pass straight into the dorsal columns to the dorsal column nuclei. However, they first send important collaterals into laminae III, IV and V of the dorsal horn (Figure 3.5).

These activate interneurones which secrete γ-amino butyric acid (GABA) which inhibits transmission of nociceptive impulses in SG cells. Thus, stroking or rubbing can relieve pain segmentally, and can be imitated by TENS.

Dorsal column nuclei project to the thalamus (ventrobasal nucleus), thence to the primary and secondary sensory areas on the cortex on the same side. Dorsal column nuclei also project to the posterior nuclei of the thalamus and to the mid-brain reticular formation and its descending inhibitory control, explaining the analgesia produced by dorsal column stimulation.

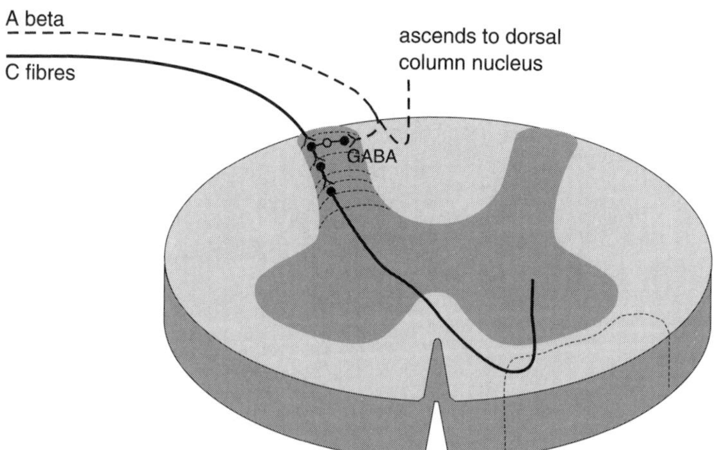

Figure 3.5 Probable mechanism of transcutaneous electrical nerve stimulation (TENS). Diagram of spinal cord showing pathway of A beta fibres into dorsal column; collaterals pass into dorsal horn to activate GABA interneurone and thereby inhibit the substantia gelatinosa cells.

Descending inhibition

As we have seen, stimulating A delta afferents eventually activates the hypothalamus (arcuate nucleus). This in turn activates descending chain reactions, which inhibit nociception throughout the spinal cord. There are probably several descending inhibitory systems, of which two are well defined (Takashige *et al.*, 1992, 1993), as shown diagrammatically in Figure 3.6. One route is a serotonin-mediated pathway, which involves midline structures, the periaqueductal grey (PAG) and the nucleus raphe magnus (nRM). The other route is the noradrenaline-mediated pathway, which descends either side of the midline, through the gigantocellular and paragigantocellular nuclei.

Serotoninergic system

The PAG is central to the serotoninergic pathway: electrical stimulation of the PAG produced sufficient analgesia to permit abdominal surgery in rats, and the PAG is the area of the brain where the smallest dose of morphine causes the greatest analgesia (Bowsher, 1998). Stimulating electrodes implanted into the PAG in chronic pain patients produces pain relief which is reversed by naloxone, although this reversal has been challenged (Young and Chambi, 1987).

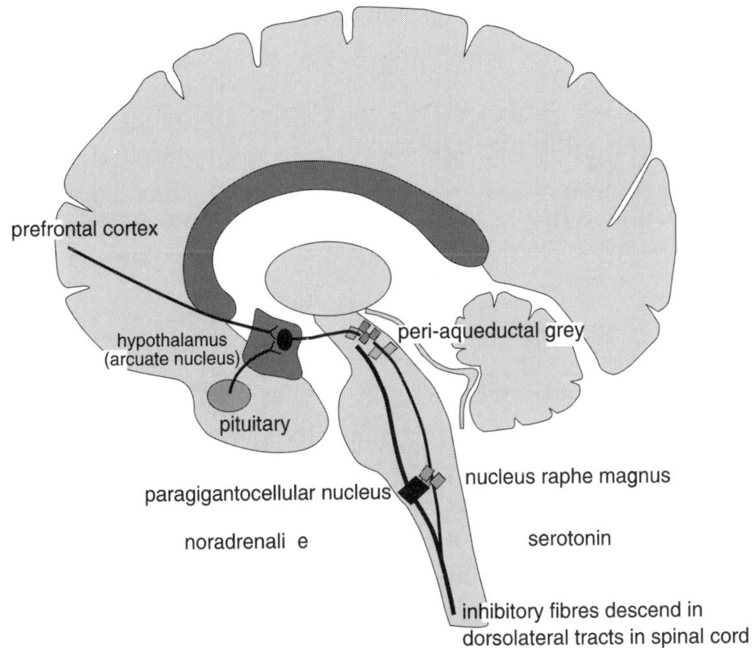

Figure 3.6 Diagram of sagittal section of the brain showing probable origin of descending inhibitory systems. The prefrontal cortex and pituitary stimulate the hypothalamus (arcuate nucleus) to activate the periaqueductal grey. From there, two descending systems are shown: midline serotonergic system, involving the raphe magnus: and noradrenergic system either side of the midline involving the paragigantocellular nucleus.

The PAG activates the nRM from which axons travel in the dorsolateral columns to dorsal horns throughout the spinal cord. The fibres terminate on laminae I, II and V, also on the ventral horn and sympathetic and parasympathetic cell columns. They release serotonin that activates 'stalked' cells at the junction of laminae I and II, leading to the release of enkephalin which inhibits the SG cells (Figure 3.7).

The arcuate nucleus of the hypothalamus, the PAG and the nRM have close reciprocal connections with the prefrontal cortex, the hypothalamus, septum and limbic system and are probably sites where the perception of pain can be influenced by emotional and other psychological factors such as attention and memory.

Noradrenergic system

The parallel descending inhibitory system is less well understood: the hypothalamus (arcuate nucleus) activates the gigantocellular and paragigantocellular nuclei of the brainstem; the locus coeruleus of the pons is also implicated. Descending inhibitory fibres again travel in the dorsolateral columns. These release noradrenaline diffusely through the dorsal horn, directly inhibiting SG cells (Figure 3.7).

Thus we see the complete loop of nociceptive control: the A delta afferent pathway ends in the hypothalamus and activates the descending inhibitory pathway. It is interesting to note that the nRM retains somatotopic representation, and Bowsher (1998) has hypothesized that this may be the basis for the strong effect of certain acupuncture points on pain.

Diffuse noxious inhibitory control

Another mechanism of analgesia involves a noxious stimulus anywhere in the body, and is known as diffuse noxious inhibitory control (DNIC). Le Bars *et al.* (1979) recorded directly from convergent cells in the lumbar

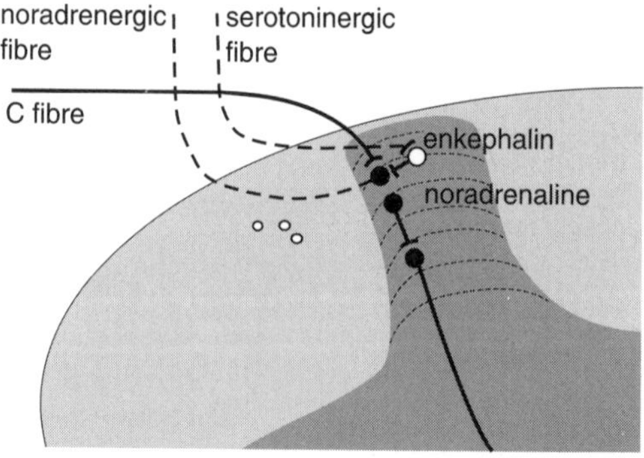

Figure 3.7 Action of descending inhibitory systems at the spinal cord level: serotoninergic fibres activate interneurones to release enkephalin. Noradrenergic fibres release noradrenaline to diffuse through the dorsal horn. Both mechanisms inhibit transmission of nociceptive impulses through the substantia gelatinosa.

region of intact anaesthetized rats, observing the cells' response to C fibre stimulation. This response was inhibited by noxious stimulation at any site, including tail, muzzle, paws or viscera, and by any modality, including pinch, electrical stimulation, heat or bradykinin. Innocuous stimulation had no effect. Inhibition sometimes lasted two and a half times the duration of the noxious stimulus. The mechanism of DNIC involves supraspinal loops (Le Bars and Willer, 1988). It has been suggested that DNIC may heighten the contrast between neuronal responses to background stimulation and a noxious event, increasing the likelihood of the appreciation of injury (Le Bars *et al.*, 1979). This phenomenon explains why patients with chronic pain have a higher pain tolerance than normal volunteers (Le Bars and Willer, 1988).

Further inhibitory mechanisms are likely to be discovered: for example, Sandkuhler *et al.* (1996) presented evidence suggesting that propriospinal systems may be an important component of nociceptive control.

Neurotransmitters and acupuncture

Acupuncture analgesia was shown to depend on a humoral mechanism (Research Group of Acupuncture Anaesthesia, 1974). Cerebrospinal fluid (CSF) was removed from a rabbit in which acupuncture analgesia had been induced. This donor CSF was used to replace the CSF of a recipient rabbit, which in turn developed analgesia. The important questions are whether this finding is relevant to clinical acupuncture in humans, and which components of the CSF were responsible for transmitting the analgesia. Several candidates will be discussed here.

Opioid peptides

Opioid peptides and their receptors are widely distributed in the CNS, particularly in relation to known nociceptive pathways. Three opioid peptides are known to be involved in analgesia: **enkephalins** are present in laminae I and V of the dorsal horn and the PAG; **beta-endorphin** is found in the PAG and the arcuate nucleus of the hypothalamus; **dynorphin** is found throughout the spinal cord. Opioid peptides produce their effect after binding to receptor sites, of which three types (mu, kappa and delta) have been identified. Each receptor is stimulated preferentially by one of the peptides, though not exclusively. Opioid receptors are present either side of the C fibre synapse in the substantia gelatinosa. Presynaptically, receptor activation may block Ca^{2+} channels, thus preventing transmitter release. Postsynaptically, receptor activation may increase the action of the K^+ pump, increasing the membrane's resting potential and thus stabilizing it against depolarization. The analgesic effects of opioid peptides are powerful, as shown by the profound analgesia resulting when beta-endorphin is administered intrathecally (Oyama *et al.*, 1980).

Opioid peptides are not only released within the CNS, but also secreted into the bloodstream from the pituitary gland. This involves the breakdown of the precursor, proopiocortin, into beta-endorphin and ACTH, which are released in parallel. Opioid peptide concentrations in the blood increase in association with a number of stimuli including stress, physical exercise, sex and conditioning (Hawkes, 1992). However, they are not likely to generate central analgesia because they cannot readily cross the blood–brain barrier. Concentrations of opioid peptides cannot be directly correlated with the level of analgesia. For example, Moret *et al.* (1991), exploring the use of acupuncture for surgical analgesia, found that pre-injection of hydrocortisone prevented any rise in the plasma concentration of beta-endorphin but did not affect the level of analgesia.

Professor Han's laboratory in Beijing has been one of the foremost in unravelling the role of opioid peptides in acupuncture analgesia and the early work has been summarized (Han and Terenius, 1982). The key findings were that low frequency EA triggers the release of beta-endorphin and enkephalin in the brain and spinal cord, which interact with mu and delta receptors respectively. By contrast, high-frequency (or 'TENS-like') EA increases the release of dynorphin in the spinal cord, which interacts with kappa receptors. These findings have been confirmed in humans (Han *et al.*, 1991).

Critical studies showed that acupuncture analgesia (AA) is inhibited by microinjection of naloxone into many areas of the brain, particularly the PAG; and that D-phenylalanine or D-leucine, which inhibit opioid degradation enzymes, potentiate the analgesic effects of AA without themselves causing any increase in analgesia (Cheng and Pomeranz 1980; Ehrenpreis, 1985).

The existence of antagonists specific to different receptors has been crucial in elucidating the role of neurotransmitters. For example, most studies conclude that naloxone, which specifically binds to the mu receptor, reverses low-frequency analgesia (Pomeranz and Cheng, 1979). Naloxone and other specific antagonists were used by Chen *et al.* (1996) to demonstrate that analgesia induced by 2-Hz stimulation involves both mu and delta receptors; analgesia induced by 30-Hz stimulation is mediated by all three opioid receptor types; and analgesia induced by 100-Hz stimulation is mediated primarily by kappa receptors.

The role of opioid peptides in AA has not gone unchallenged. Bossut *et al.* (1991) replicated Han's experiments with acupuncture stimulation and found considerable discrepancies. The level of analgesia produced by acupuncture in these experiments in the USA was considerably lower than that obtained by Han and colleagues in China. Naloxone not only failed to reverse the analgesia induced by low-frequency EA, but actually potentiated the analgesia induced by high-frequency EA. The response to acupuncture altered with exposure: naloxone increased analgesia in acupuncture-naïve animals, but reversed analgesia in animals that had been pre-exposed to acupuncture more than once (Bossut and Mayer, 1991b). The authors concluded that the analgesic response changes considerably with conditioning to the environment; opioid peptides are neither sufficient to explain acupuncture analgesia, nor indeed essential to the phenomenon.

Cholecystokinin

One puzzling aspect of nociceptive control is that the stimulus that provokes the release of opioid peptides also provokes the release of an antagonist to them, cholecystokinin (CCK). Han *et al.* (1986a) found that CCK injected into either the cerebral ventricles or the spinal cord abolished AA. Release of CCK requires 2 hours' continuous stimulation, although less if the stimulation is stopped and repeated within a short period. It seems that nociceptive control may represent a balance between opioid peptide activity and CCK activity. It is not known whether the actions of CCK are relevant to the acupuncture tolerance which occurs with repeated use of acupuncture clinically.

Serotonin (5-hydroxytryptamine, 5HT)

Han and Terenius (1982) summarized the evidence that serotonin is involved in AA. In animals, inhibition of serotonin synthesis produces a parallel lowering of serotonin concentration and analgesia; blockade of serotonin receptors reduces analgesia. Loading animals with serotonin precursor, or blocking serotonin degradation, potentiate analgesia. In humans, the effect of the tricyclic drug clomipramine (which blocks serotonin reuptake from nerve terminals) on acupressure analgesia was tested in a randomized controlled trial: clomipramine increased the analgesic effect of acupressure ('finger-pressing anaesthesia') for extraction of impacted third molar teeth. The study was published in Chinese (Zhao *et al.*, 1978).

Oxytocin

Oxytocin is released centrally in response to suckling. Oxytocin administered to rats causes analgesia. Interestingly, oxytocin may have a role in background analgesia, because blockade of oxytocin receptors lowers the pain threshold in normal rats. Uvnas-Moburg *et al.* (1993) detected increases in oxytocin in both plasma and CSF after electrical stimulation at 2 Hz, as well as warmth and high-frequency vibration. Analgesia as assessed by tail-flick latency increased in parallel, and was reversed by receptor blockade but not naloxone.

Evidence for the effect of acupuncture on acute pain: human research

Evidence of acupuncture's effects on pain in humans consists of direct observation of change in pain threshold, and indirect evidence from neurotransmitter activity.

Changes in pain threshold

In an early systematic study of acupuncture analgesia, Chiang *et al.* (1973) explored the effect of acupuncture on pain threshold in a series of experiments with 21 human volunteers. Acupuncture needles in the hand were stimulated (in the authors' own words) 'by a mechanical acupuncture manipulator which acted at a frequency of 2/s, with a moving distance of 3.0–5.5 mm and a twirling angle of 90–165° depending on the individual tolerance'. By any standards, this was a remarkably strong stimulation. After 16 minutes, pain thresholds to electric current increased significantly at various points of the body. In a subsequent experiment, local anaesthetic or saline was injected into the muscle beneath the acupuncture point before needling; local anaesthetic, but not saline, inhibited the analgesic effect.

Andersson *et al.* (1973) were the first western authors to report analgesia in humans after EA. Eighteen dental student volunteers received electrostimulation to a pair of needles, one in the hand and one in the face near the infraorbital nerve. Analgesia was assessed by measuring the threshold to electrical stimulation of dental pulp: the threshold gradually rose over 30 minutes, then slowly decayed after stimulation was ended. However, there are several aspects of this study which make its results less impressive. First, it was uncontrolled and does not allow for placebo effects. Second, the method of measuring dental pulp pain was not rigorous and current leakage across damp teeth may have exaggerated the effect. Third, the degree of stimulation was extremely strong and too painful to use in chronic pain patients (Sjolund and Eriksson, 1979).

Systematic review: manual acupuncture

Clearly, reliable evidence of the existence of acupuncture analgesia phenomenon relies on blinded, controlled trials in which subjects receive either genuine or indistinguishable sham acupuncture.

Systematic searches of Medline and CISCOM databases were used to locate controlled studies of manual acupuncture (MA) and EA for experimental analgesia. Table 3.2 gives details of all 12 trials of MA that were located.

In all but two studies, the control procedure was needling of off-site off-meridian locations. In the study reported by Chiang *et al.* (1973), controls received injection of local anaesthetic (as above); the study by Mayer *et al.* (1977) was rather different in that subjects who experienced analgesia were then injected with either naloxone or saline in a double-blind fashion. The overall result of the review provides no support for an analgesic effect of MA. There is no evidence that the result would have been any different by isolating one aspect of acupuncture technique (such as number of needles, duration of needling, strength of stimulation), or one particular type of test pain. The balance of evidence is not in support of either a segmental or an extrasegmental effect.

However, there are problems with the reliability of the evidence. Three studies (Smith *et al.*, 1974; Li *et al.*, 1975; Saletu *et al.*, 1975) showed positive trends with small samples, and may conceal type II errors. Because the response to acupuncture differs greatly between individual subjects, a large sample size may be required to show a significant effect unless 'responders' are preselected for the study (Chapman *et al.*, 1983).

Table 3.2 Controlled trials of manual acupuncture for experimental pain. (Positive studies = acupuncture sig. better than control; negative studies = no sig. difference.)

First author	*Year*	*Design*	*n (treatment, control)*	*Number of needles*	*Strength of stimulation*[1]	*Type of test pain*	*Pain site*[2]
Positive studies							
Chiang	1973	crossover	21	2	3	electrical	E
Stacher	1975	crossover	12	2	3	electrical	E
Umlauf	1976	parallel	(12,12)	2	3	electrical	E
Mayer	1977	parallel	(9,11)[3]	2	2	electrical	E
Lundeberg[4]	1989	crossover	6	2	2	electrical	S
Brockhaus	1990	parallel	(25,15)	2	1	heat	S
Negative studies							
Smith	1974	crossover	15	6	3	ischaemia	S
Li	1975	crossover	14	1–5	2	electrical	E
Saletu	1975	crossover	20	2	?	electrical	S
Boureau	1978	crossover	10	1	?	nociceptive reflex	E
Lundeberg[4]	1989	crossover	6	2	2	electrical	E
Johnson	1996	parallel	(6,6,6)	1	2	electrical	S

[1]Manipulation score: 0 = none; 1 = on insertion only; 2 = repeated intermittent; 3 = continuous.
[2]S = segmental; E = extrasegmental.
[3]Preselected by good response to acupuncture.
[4]Two studies published in one report.

Responders comprise only 57% (Mayer *et al.*, 1977) or 42% (Chapman *et al.*, 1983) of healthy volunteers.

In summary, the evidence as it stands does not demonstrate convincingly that manual acupuncture produces analgesia reliably in humans.

Systematic review: electroacupuncture

The search for studies of electroacupuncture for experimental pain located 12 reports of controlled trials with data presented in a usable form, which are listed in Table 3.3.

In contrast to the evidence on MA, the weight of evidence is in favour of a conclusion that EA produces analgesia in humans. Of the four negative studies, those reported by Pauser *et al.* (1975) and Smith *et al.* (1974) showed trends in favour of an acupuncture effect. It is interesting to note that the high-frequency (TENS-like) stimulation was effective in every case where it was used, whereas studies that used low-frequency (acupuncture-like) stimulation were equally divided between positive and negative.

The combined evidence does not throw any light on the question of whether there is a difference between segmental and extrasegmental effects. However, parallel studies by Lundeberg *et al.* (1989) found that dental analgesia could be produced by local segmental needling in the face, but not by extrasegmental needling using points in the hand.

Table 3.3 Controlled trials of electroacupuncture *vs* sham acupuncture for experimental pain. (Positive studies = acupuncture sig. better than control; negative studies = no sig. difference.)

First author	*Year*	*Design*	*n (treatment, control)*	*Number of needles*	*Frequency of stimulation (Hz)*	*Type of test pain*	*Pain site*[1]
Positive studies							
Anderson	1974	parallel	(10,10)	4	?	cold pressor	S
Berlin	1975	parallel	(10,10)	2	120	radiant heat	S
Saletu	1975	crossover	20	2	130	elec-current	S
Chapman	1976	parallel	(15,15)	2	2	dental pulp	E
Stern	1977	crossover	20	4	130	cold pressor	S
Stewart	1977	crossover	12	2	2.5	radiant heat	E
Boureau	1978	crossover	10	1	500	nociceptive reflex	E
Chapman	1980	parallel	(10,10)	1	2	dental pulp	E
Lundeberg[2]	1989	crossover	6	2	2	dental pulp	S
Negative studies							
Pauser	1973	crossover	16	5	3	pressure	E
Smith	1974	crossover	10	6	?	ischaemia	S
Knox[3]	1979	crossover	24	2	3	cold pressor	S
Lundeberg[2]	1989	crossover	6	2	2	dental pulp	E

[1]S = segmental; E = extrasegmental.
[2]Two studies published in one report.
[3]Knox (1979): positive result for subgroup of subjects with high expectancy.

Thus, it appears that EA does have a genuine analgesic effect in humans. How large is that effect? It was not possible to calculate formal effect sizes (i.e. change in endpoint divided by standard deviation) because too few authors reported standard deviations. Therefore, the percentage change in the endpoint of each study was converted into the equivalent increase in threshold, a method that ignores the distribution about the mean and is therefore subject to error. Reports by Pauser *et al.* (1975), Smith *et al.* (1974) and Chapman *et al.* (1980) were omitted, as they did not include appropriate data. Figure 3.8 shows the results for the remaining nine studies. As shown in Figure 3.8, most studies found that acupuncture raised the threshold by about 20–30%, too small to be useful clinically. Similar conversion of results of other controlled trials show that acupuncture is a less potent analgesic than hypnosis (Figure 3.9), and about the same potency as various analgesics with which it was compared (Figure 3.10).

Clinical pain

Obviously, the evidence of effectiveness of acupuncture in experimental pain does not necessarily translate directly to clinical pain (Woolf, 1979; Gracely, 1991). The effect of acupuncture on pre-existing clinical pain was investigated by searching our own files for relevant studies. The five

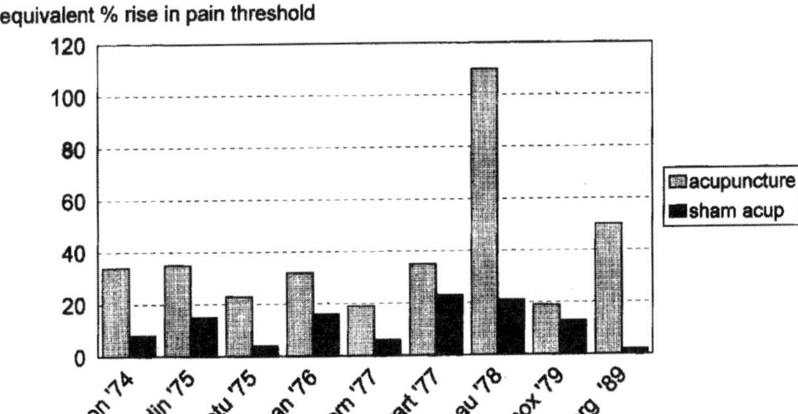

Figure 3.8 Analgesia to experimental pain produced by electroacupuncture and sham electroacupuncture in nine controlled trials. Results have been converted into an equivalent percentage rise in pain threshold; see text for the limitations of this method.

studies located (Table 3.4) form a rather heterogeneous group in terms of condition treated, control used and endpoint.

Three studies found that acupuncture had a significant effect on the pain; two were negative but showed trends in the same direction. Thus, there is rather flimsy evidence in favour of a short-term effect of acupuncture on painful clinical conditions.

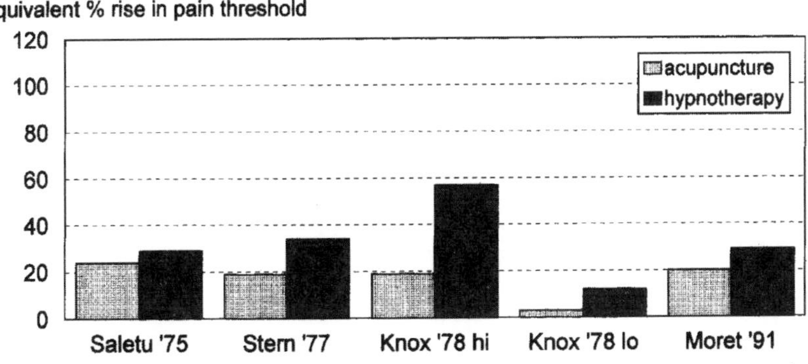

Figure 3.9 Electroacupuncture analgesia compared with hypnotherapy analgesia for experimental pain. Results have been converted into equivalent percentage rise in pain threshold; see text for limitations of this method. Note: hi and lo indicate subjects with high or low hypnotic susceptibility.

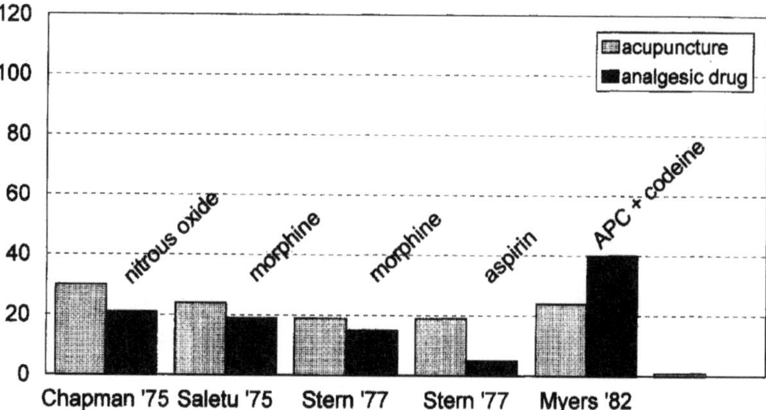

Figure 3.10 Electroacupuncture analgesia compared with various pharmaceutical analgesics for experimental pain. Results have been converted into equivalent percentage rise in pain threshold; see text for limitations of this method.

Neurotransmitter activity

Reversal by naloxone

An integral component of the opioid peptide hypothesis is the ability of naloxone to reverse analgesia. Mayer *et al.* (1977) selected 20 out of 31 volunteers who responded well to acupuncture. Needles were inserted into both hands and manipulated manually for 2 minutes every 5 minutes over the following half hour. The pain threshold, measured by electrical stimulation of dental pulp, increased by an average 27% after acupuncture. The subjects were then given an injection of either 0.8 mg naloxone or an equal volume of saline, in a double-blind fashion. The pain threshold in the naloxone group fell virtually to pre-test levels, whereas that of the saline group showed no change.

Chapman *et al.* (1980) planned to replicate Mayer's experiment but found that the manual stimulation technique was too painful for the subjects; needles were therefore stimulated electrically. The resulting analgesia, as measured by brain-evoked potentials, was not reversed by naloxone. This work was criticized by Mayer and Price (1981) because brain-evoked potentials may not truly reflect pain sensation, and because the dose of naloxone was inadequate, i.e. 0.4 mg. Chapman and colleagues repeated the study correcting these issues (Chapman *et al.*, 1983). Fourteen subjects who responded to acupuncture were given low-frequency EA for 30 minutes. Analgesia, this time measured by dental pulp threshold, rose by an average of 30%. The subjects then received either 1.2 mg naloxone or saline, chosen at random. There was a small reversal in the analgesia after naloxone, which did not reach statistical significance. These authors concluded that their own work and other studies 'provided little convincing evidence that endorphins play a significant role in acupunctural analgesia' (Chapman *et al.*, 1983).

Table 3.4 Controlled studies of the short-term effect of acupuncture (manual or electrical) on pre-existing clinical pain

First author	*Year*	*Condition*	*No.*	*Control*	*Endpoint*	*Pain relief*		*P value*
						Acupuncture	*Control*	
Lundeberg	1984	myalgia	36	sugar pill	50% relief	22/36	10/36	<0.01
Lundeberg *et al.*	1988a	sinus pain	35	superficial acup.	50% relief	13/21	5/21	<0.05
Lundeberg *et al.*	1991	neck pain	58	superficial acup.	pain relief	35%	21%	NS
Thomas *et al.*	1991	neck pain	44	superficial acup.	pain relief	28%	20%	NS
Molsberger and Hille	1994	lateral epicondylitis	94	sham stimulation	mean pain relief	56%	15%	<0.01

acup. = acupuncture; NS = not significant.

Table 3.5 Controlled trials of double-blind injection of naloxone vs saline in attempt to reverse electroacupuncture analgesia

First author	*Year*	*Design*	*n (treatment, control)*	*Number of needles*	*Frequency of stimulation (Hz)*	*Type of test pain*	*Pain site*[1]	*Result*
Boureau	1979	parallel	8[2]	2	2	nociceptive reflex, supraorbital nerve	E	positive $P<0.001$
Chapman	1983	parallel	(7,7)[2]	2	2	electrical dental pulp	E	negative
Ernst	1987	crossover	5	1	2	electrical dental pulp	E	positive $P<0.005$
Lundeberg	1989	crossover	6	2	2, 80[3]	electrical dental pulp	S	negative
Moret	1991	crossover	8	2	130	cold pressor	S	negative

[1]S = segmental; E = extrasegmental.

[2]Selected good responders.

[3]Separate studies with 2 and 80 Hz had similar results.

The systematic literature search performed above located five controlled trials in which investigators compared naloxone and saline for reversal of EA analgesia (Table 3.5).

Unfortunately, all trials have small sample sizes. Two studies were positive, three were negative. This supports the conclusion of Chapman *et al.* (1983) that EA analgesia does not depend exclusively on opioid peptide release.

CSF opioid concentrations

Clement-Jones *et al.* (1980) were the first to show that CSF beta-endorphin concentrations rise after EA. Beta-endorphin levels rose significantly in ten subjects with pain relief but not in eight untreated controls who had no pain relief. Met-enkephalin concentrations in CSF did not change in either group. Similar changes were observed by Zhang *et al.* (1980). Sjolund *et al.* (1977) also detected a rise in CSF beta-endorphin after acupuncture-like TENS. Han *et al.* (1991) showed that low- and high-frequency electrical stimulation release different opioid peptides in the CNS. Patients who were about to receive routine lumbar punctures for other reasons were randomized to receive either 2-Hz or 100-Hz TENS for 30 minutes before a second CSF sample was taken. 2-Hz stimulation led to a significant increase of met-enkephalin but not dynorphin A, whereas 100-Hz stimulation produced a significant increase in dynorphin A but not met-enkephalin.

However, the concentration of neurotransmitters in the CSF does not necessarily reflect their activity within the spinal cord, and can at best provide circumstantial evidence of their role in pain relief.

Evidence for the effect of acupuncture on acute pain: animal research

A variety of experiments with animals has helped to elucidate both the pathways and the mechanisms of nociceptive control. There have been two general approaches. First, **functional anatomy** can be explored by cutting tracts or ablating nuclei to observe the effect on analgesia, or by stimulating particular sites and searching for electrical responses or biochemical changes elsewhere. Second, the effect of acupuncture on **neurotransmitters** has been explored through direct measurement of concentrations, or through observing the effect of manipulating neurotransmitter activity. The overall evidence for involvement of endogenous opioid peptides has been reviewed above, and here we are concerned with their role in different parts of the CNS involved with descending inhibitory control.

Acupuncture and the spinal cord

Pomeranz and Cheng (1979) recorded directly from single cells in the lamina V of the cat dorsal horn; low-frequency EA inhibited the response to a nociceptive stimulus by about 20% in the same segment, but not the response to touch. Analgesia reached a maximum after 20 minutes and slowly declined after the end of stimulation. This analgesia was abolished in spinalized animals, indicating that the analgesic effect of EA involves supraspinal centres in cats.

In order to investigate the segmental effect of acupuncture, Chung *et al.* (1984) made similar direct intracellular recordings from cells in the lamina V of monkey dorsal horn. They recorded the discharges evoked by C fibre stimulation of the sural nerve repeated every 10 seconds. The response of the lamina V cells was isolated from descending influence of the brainstem by using spinalized animal preparations. The lamina V cell responses were completely inhibited within minutes of starting 2-Hz electrostimulation of nearby peripheral nerves. The effect was greatest when the electrostimulation was given in adjacent segments, and diminished progressively with stimulation of the contralateral limb, the upper limb on the same side, and the upper limb on the other side. Further experiments revealed that the strength of the inhibition increased as the frequency of stimulation increased from 0.5 to 20 Hz. The analgesia was only partially reversed by naloxone. Because this analgesia occurred in spinal animals, it depends, at least in part, on local spinal cord circuitry.

Acupuncture and the ascending arm of the inhibitory loop

The fact that the ascending (ventral) tracts were essential for analgesia was first demonstrated by Chiang *et al.* (1975). After sectioning these tracts in rabbits, the analgesia produced by MA to the contralateral hind limb was completely abolished. By contrast, the analgesia was completely unaffected by section of the dorsal columns.

Acupuncture and brainstem nuclei

The periaqueductal grey (PAG) is believed to be central to nociceptive control. Wang *et al.* (1990) showed that lesions of the PAG attenuated both high- and low-frequency EA analgesia. Zhang *et al.* (1980) found that EA increased the opioid content of the PAG (as well as caudate and nucleus accumbens), which correlated with the degree of inhibition of nociceptor responses. Naloxone microinjection into the PAG in rabbits reversed EA analgesia in a dose one-tenth of the dose effective by intraventricular injection, and one four hundredth the dose effective intravenously (Zhang *et al.*, 1980).

Liu *et al.* (1986), recording directly from excitatory neurones in the nucleus raphe magnus, found that EA increased their background firing rates, consistent with a role in acupuncture analgesia.

The role of the pituitary has been the subject of some discussion. Pomeranz *et al.* (1977) found that hypophysectomy reduced EA analgesia and formed an initial hypothesis that pituitary release of beta-endorphin into the bloodstream was important in AA, acting by diffusion back across the blood–brain barrier. By contrast, Bossut and Mayer (1991b) found that EA analgesia was greater in rats after hypophysectomy than in sham-operated controls. This suggests that EA analgesia is either independent of beta-endorphin released into the circulation from the pituitary, or even antagonized by it.

Further support for the hypothesis that electroacupuncture analgesia involves brainstem nuclei comes from newer techniques such as fos expression. Fos is the nuclear phosphorylation product of mammalian C-*fos* proto-oncogene. It is induced by nerve stimulation, as well as by nerve growth factor and cholinergic transmitters. C-*fos* is detected by immunocytochemical methods after sacrifice of the animal and therefore acts as a short-term marker for neuronal activation (Lee and Beitz, 1993). However, care is needed in interpreting the results of studies, because not all neurones are able to induce C-*fos*, and C-*fos* is expressed strongly in several areas of the brainstem in response to non-specific stimuli such as transport and handling.

Lee and Beitz (1993) and Guo *et al.* (1996) found that low-frequency and high-frequency EA in rats induced patterns of C-*fos* expression which were similar in many brainstem nuclei including the PAG. Low-frequency EA activated some areas which were not activated by high-frequency EA, which the authors suggested was related to naloxone reversibility. Many other areas of telencephalon, diencephalon and mid brainstem showed significant increases in C-*fos* expression after EA compared with manual needling or no treatment controls. Stimulation of non-acupuncture points did not produce significant C-*fos* expression (Lee and Beitz, 1993).

Guo *et al.* (1996) used a special technique (in situ hybridization) that detects changes in the messenger RNA molecules that code for the different opioid precursors. Electroacupuncture at 2-Hz induced the expression of **preproenkephalin** mRNA in particular, mainly in the arcuate nucleus, the paraventricular hypothalamic nucleus and the ventral nucleus of the lateral lemniscus. On the other hand, 100-Hz EA was accompanied by a significant increase in **preprodynorphin**, the principal sites being the supraoptic, paraventricular hypothalamic, ventromedial and lateral parabrachial nuclei. Neither frequency affected the proopiomelanocortin mRNA. This suggests that EA may result in changes in the genetic expression of neurotransmitters. If confirmed, this could provide an explanation for the sustained effects of acupuncture observed clinically.

Acupuncture and the descending (inhibitory) arm

Shen and colleagues (1978) demonstrated that the descending arm of the loop was essential for AA. Using intact anaesthetized cats, these workers measured the cortical-evoked potential from noxious stimulation applied to the splanchnic nerve. This response was inhibited by EA to the hind leg; however, cutting the dorsolateral fibres of the spinal cord at T3 segmental level prevented the effect of the EA. To address the criticism that this transection might cut the ascending arm of the inhibitory loop, they repeated the experiment stimulating the forepaw, i.e. above the level of spinal cord section. Analgesia was again inhibited by transection of the dorsolateral tracts, confirming the role of these descending fibres.

Han *et al.* (1982) measured analgesia simultaneously in head and tail of rabbits during acupuncture stimulation. Injection of antiserum against enkephalins into the spinal cord inhibited analgesia locally, i.e. in the tail, but not in the head. A similar result was obtained by Han *et al.* (1984) with anti-dynorphin, suggesting that the descending arm of analgesia involves both these neurotransmitters.

Bing *et al.* (1991) measured the ability of MA to release met-enkephalin in the rat spinal cord. CSF was collected from the thoracic and lumbar areas separately in anaesthetized animals during 15-minute periods of stimulation of either a recognized acupuncture point (ST 36) or a nearby non-point. Needling at the acupuncture point produced 10 minutes' significant rise in the release of met-enkephalin in the thoracic cord, though not the lumbar cord (i.e. heterosegmental but not segmental effect). Needling of the non-acupuncture point was also followed by the release of opioid peptide in this study, whereas it did not lead to C-*fos* expression in a subsequent study (Lee and Beitz, 1993).

Thus we have seen that there is reasonable evidence from a variety of experimental models in different centres that acupuncture (mainly electroacupuncture) can modulate nociception. Some of the mechanisms are understood in considerable detail.

Problems and future directions

Manual versus electroacupuncture

It seems unlikely that a single mechanism could explain the effects of EA and MA. They are different clinically: MA produces at most a brief muscle contraction, and a discharge of A delta nerves that lasts for only a few minutes after the end of stimulation (Wang *et al.*, 1985). By contrast, EA is aimed at achieving regular, continuous stimulation of nerve fibres from muscle for 10–20 minutes accompanied by visible muscle contraction. Although both methods of stimulation may activate predominantly A delta fibres, it cannot be assumed that the central response is identical, given the complexities of sensory information coding, neuronal connections, differences in accommodation and refractory periods of dorsal horn cells, and duration of afterdischarges in various components of the CNS.

Moreover, there is positive evidence that MA and EA have significantly different effects. For example, Dawidson *et al.* (1997) showed clearly that salivary flow rate increased with MA but not with EA; Saletu *et al.* (1975) found that EA and MA generated different EEG responses; Nappi *et al.* (1982) found that EA released beta-endorphin and ACTH into the plasma, whereas MA released beta-endorphin but not ACTH. The duration of release of beta-endorphin and beta-lipotropin was much shorter after MA than EA. Bucinskaite *et al.* (1994) compared the effects of MA, EA, superficial needling and exercise on rat CNS neuropeptides. Electroacupuncture increased the concentrations of vasoactive intestinal peptide (VIP) in striatum, neuropeptide Y in the hippocampus and occipital cortex, and substance P and neurokinin A in the hippocampus. MA performed once or ten times, and a single running exercise, had no effect on any of these neuropeptides tested.

It does not seem justified to assume that the results of research into EA are necessarily directly relevant to normal clinical practice, which usually involves manual stimulation of needles.

The problem of acupuncture points

This is still an unresolved issue. On the one hand, there are a number of studies which show that acupuncture is more effective when it is given at recognized acupuncture points than random points; see, for example, the summary of EA for experimental pain above. Furthermore, traditional acupuncture theory holds that particular acupuncture points not only exist, but have specific functions, and there is evidence in support of this (e.g. Vickers, 1996). On the other hand, many clinicians have given up using standard points and traditional theory altogether, without apparently loss of clinical effect (see Chapter 2). It is to be hoped that modern methods of investigation such as MRI (Cho *et al.*, 1998), transcranial Doppler sonography (Litscher *et al.*, 1997) or positron emission scintography (Jones *et al.*, 1991), will resolve these issues.

Sustained effects of acupuncture

In the majority of experiments of AA in animals, nociception returns to normal about 20 minutes after the end of stimulation. However, clinical experience suggests that the effect of acupuncture lasts much longer than 20 minutes. Vierck *et al.* (1974) found sustained behavioural changes, compatible with analgesia, in monkeys up to 70 hours after EA. Price *et al.* (1984) also found both a delayed onset of analgesia (1–24 hours) in some patients with pain, and an effect prolonged for 10–14 days. Unfortunately, the importance of these two studies is limited because they were uncontrolled. If the mechanisms of acute analgesia have not been established unequivocally after 20 years, there seems little hope of early solutions to the problems of delayed or sustained analgesia.

Possible mechanisms that have been suggested for sustained analgesia include the mesolimbic loop of Han *et al.* (1986b), long-term depression of the superficial spinal horn by low-frequency stimulation of afferent A fibres (Sandkuhler *et al.*, 1996) and induction of mRNA for opioid peptide expression (Guo *et al.*, 1996).

Variation in response to acupuncture

Humans and animals share one interesting feature, viz. marked individual variation in response to acupuncture. This is clearly reported in humans (Mayer *et al.*, 1977; Chapman *et al.*, 1983) and in rats (Bossut *et al.*, 1991).

It has been suggested that this variation in response might be affected by dietary intake of D-phenylalanine and D-leucine. The effect of acupuncture on experimental pain (mouse vocalization model) is augmented in mice which have been pre-treated with the D-amino acids (Cheng and Pomeranz, 1980). Takeshige *et al.* (1993) recorded directly the mouse PAG response to EA stimulation of the tibialis muscle. The PAG discharge seen in non-responders was considerably smaller than that seen in responders; it was increased after administration of D-phenylalanine. Another possible explanation involves the opioid antagonist CCK. Tang *et al.* (1997) produced evidence that non-responders had higher levels of CCK than responders, suggesting that the response to acupuncture may depend on the balance of CCK and opioid activity in the ascending arm of the inhibitory loop.

Effect of repetition of acupuncture (conditioning)

Laboratory investigations of acupuncture usually involve one-off treatment. There is some evidence that acupuncture produces a different physiological response upon repetition. For example, Bossut and Mayer (1991a) showed that acupuncture-naïve rats given EA developed analgesia that was enhanced by naloxone; it was only when acupuncture had been given several times that the better-known picture emerged of analgesia that was reversed by naloxone. Similar affects have been suggested in humans: Dyrehag *et al.* (1997) found that the first session of acupuncture produced increased sympathetic activity, whereas after a course of acupuncture sympathetic activity was decreased. The experiment was uncontrolled, so the changes could have been caused by other factors such as familiarization with the testing procedure. Han (1997) reported work which suggested that rats given acupuncture every fourth day showed gradually strengthening analgesia and increase in monoamines in the spinal perfusate. Rats given acupuncture daily showed gradual tolerance to acupuncture.

Conclusion

Electrical stimulation of nerves via acupuncture needles is capable of producing analgesia in a variety of species of animal. This model has been used in a large number of elegant experiments, which have provided good evidence for some of the mechanisms, including activation of brainstem nuclei and descending inhibitory control systems. Experimental analgesia can also be produced in humans by acupuncture involving electrical stimulation. The evidence for an analgesic effect of manual stimulation is less clear. The short-term analgesic effect of acupuncture appears too weak to be useful clinically. Acupuncture analgesia in both animals and humans involves the release of opioid peptides, but they are not the only transmitter concerned, and may not even be the most important. Descending inhibitory control systems employ serotonin at certain stages. It does not seem probable that these short-term analgesic mechanisms will explain any prolonged effect acupuncture may have in treating clinical pain or other conditions.

Acknowledgement

I am very grateful to several colleagues who helped me with the preparation of this chapter, and particularly to Professor John Thompson, both for his excellent lectures and publications on the neurophysiology of acupuncture and TENS over many years, and for his invaluable advice on the text. Nevertheless, I am solely responsible for any errors or omissions that remain.

References

Anderson, D. G., Jamieson, J. L. and Man, S. C. (1974). Analgesic effects of acupuncture on the pain of ice water: a double-blind study. *Can. J. Psychol.*, **28,** 239–245.

Andersson, S. and Lundeberg, T. (1995). Acupuncture – from empiricism to science: functional background to acupuncture effects in pain and disease. *Med. Hypotheses*, **45,** 271–281.

Andersson, S. A., Ericson, T., Holmgren, E. and Lindqvist, G. (1973). Electro-acupuncture. Effect on pain threshold measured with electrical stimulation of teeth. *Brain Res.*, **63,** 393–396.

Baldry, P. E. (1993). *Acupuncture, Trigger Points And Musculoskeletal Pain*. Edinburgh: Churchill Livingstone.

Berlin, F. S., Bartlett, R. L. and Black, J. D. (1975). Acupuncture and placebo: effects on delaying the terminating response to a painful stimulus. *Anesthesiology*, **42,** 527–531.

Bing, Z., Cesselin, F., Bourgoin, S. *et al.* (1991). Acupuncture-like stimulation induces a heterosegmental release of Met-enkephalin-like material in the rat spinal cord. *Pain*, **47,** 71–77.

Bossut, D. F. and Mayer, D. J. (1991a). Electroacupuncture analgesia in rats: naltrexone antagonism is dependent on previous exposure. *Brain Res.*, **549,** 47–51.

Bossut, D. F. and Mayer, D. J. (1991b). Electroacupuncture analgesia in naive rats: effects of brainstem and spinal cord lesions, and role of pituitary–adrenal axis. *Brain Res.*, **549,** 52–58.

Bossut, D. F., Hung, Z. S., Sun, S. L. and Mayer, D. J. (1991). Electroacupuncture in rats: evidence for naloxone and naltrexone potentiation of analgesia. *Brain Res.*, **549,** 36–46.

Boureau, F., Sebille, A., Willer, J. C. *et al.* (1978). Effets d'une stimulation electrique heterosegmentaire percutanee (electro-acupuncture) sur le reflexe nociceptif de flexion chez l'homme. *Ann. Anesth. Franc.*, **19,** 422–426 (in French).

Boureau, F., Willer, J. C., Yamaguchi, Y. (1979). Abolition par la naloxone de l'effet inhibiteur d'une stimulation electrique peripherique sur la composante tardive du reflexe de clignement. *Electroencephalography & Clinical Neurophysiology*, **47**, 322–328.

Bowsher, D. (1987). The physiology of acupuncture. *Acupunct. Med.*, **4,** 12–14.

Bowsher, D. (1998). Mechanisms of acupuncture. In *Medical Acupuncture. A Western Scientific Approach* (J. Filshie and A. White, eds), pp. 69–82. Edinburgh: Churchill Livingstone.

Brockhaus, A. and Elger, C. E. (1990). Hypalgesic efficacy of acupuncture on experimental pain in man. Comparison of laser acupuncture and needle acupuncture. *Pain*, **43,** 181–185.

Bucinskaite, V., Lundeberg, T., Stenfors, C. *et al.* (1994). Effects of electro-acupuncture and physical exercise on regional concentrations of neuropeptides in rat brain. *Brain Res.*, **666,** 128–132.

Chan, S. H. H. (1984). What is being stimulated in acupuncture: evaluation of the existence of a specific substrate. *Neurosci. Behav. Rev.*, **8,** 25–33.

Chapman, C. R., Gehrig, J. D. and Wilson, M. E. (1975). Acupuncture compared with 33 per cent nitrous oxide for dental analgesia: a sensory decision theory evaluation. *Anesthesiology*, **42,** 532–537.

Chapman, C. R., Wilson, M. E. and Gehrig, J. D. (1976). Comparative effects of acupuncture and transcutaneous stimulation on the perception of painful dental stimuli. *Pain*, **2,** 265–283.

Chapman, C. R., Colpitts, Y., Benedetti, C. *et al.* (1980). Evoked potential assessment of acupunctural analgesia: attempted reversal with naloxone. *Pain*, **9,** 183–197.

Chapman, C. R., Benedetti, C., Colpitts, Y. H. and Gerlach, R. (1983). Naloxone fails to reverse pain thresholds elevated by acupuncture: acupuncture analgesia reconsidered. *Pain*, **16**, 13–31.

Chen, X.-H., Geller, E. B. and Adler, M. W. (1996). Electrical stimulation at traditional acupuncture sites in periphery produces brain opioid-receptor-mediated antinociception in rats. *J. Pharmacol. Exp. Ther.*, **277**, 654–660.

Cheng, R. S. S. and Pomeranz, B. (1980). A combined treatment with D-amino acids and electroacupuncture produces a greater analgesia than either treatment alone; naloxone reverses these effects. *Pain*, **8**, 231–236.

Chiang, C.-Y., Chang, C.-T., Chu, H.-L. and Yang, L.-F. (1973). Peripheral afferent pathway for acupuncture analgesia. *Sci. Sin.*, **16**, 210–217.

Chiang, C.-Y., Chu, T.-H., Liu, J.-Y. *et al.* (1975). Studies on spinal ascending pathway for effect of acupuncture analgesia in rabbits. *Sci. Sin.*, **18**, 31–34.

Cho, S-H. and Chun, S. I. (1994). The basal electrical skin resistance of acupuncture points in normal subjects. *Yonsei Med. J.*, **35**, 464–473.

Cho, Z. H., Chung, S. C., Jones, J. P. *et al.* (1998). New findings of the correlation between acupoints and corresponding brain cortices using functional MRI. *Proc. Nat. Acad. Sci. USA*, **95**, 2670–2673.

Chung, J. M., Fang, Z. R., Hori, Y. *et al.* (1984). Prolonged inhibition of primate spinothalamic tract cells by peripheral nerve stimulation. *Pain*, **19**, 259–275.

Clement-Jones, V., McLoughlin, L., Tomlin, S. *et al.* (1980). Increased beta-endorphin but not met-enkephalin levels in human cerebrospinal fluid after acupuncture for recurrent pain. *Lancet*, **316**, 945–947.

Cohen, M., Voumard, P., Birch, S. *et al.* (1995). Low resistance pathways along acupuncture meridians have dynamic behavior. *Biomed. Eng. – Applic. Basis Commun.*, **7**, 137–142.

Darras, J.-C., Albarede, P. and de Vernejoul, P. (1993). Nuclear medicine investigation of transmission of acupuncture information. *Acupunct. Med.*, **11**, 22–28.

Dawidson, I., Blom, M., Lundeberg, T. and Angmar-Mansson, B. (1997). The influence of acupuncture on salivary flow rates in healthy subjects. *J. Oral Rehabil.*, **24**, 204–208.

Dickenson, A. H. (1995). Central acute pain mechanisms. *Ann. Med.*, **27**, 223–227.

Dickenson, A. H. (1996). Pharmacology of pain transmission and control. In *Pain – An Updated Review* (J. N. Campbell, ed.). Seattle: IASP Press.

Dimond, E. G. (1971). Acupuncture anesthesia. Western medicine and Chinese traditional medicine. *JAMA*, **218**, 1558–1563.

Dung, H. C. (1984). Anatomical features contributing to the formation of acupuncture points. *Am. J. Acupunct.*, **12**, 139–143.

Dyrehag, L.-E., Widerstroem-Noga, E. G., Carlsson, S. G. and Andersson, S. A. (1997). Effects of repeated sensory stimulation sessions (electro-acupuncture) on skin temperature in chronic pain patients. *Scand. J. Rehabil. Med.*, **29**, 243–250.

Ehrenpreis, S. (1985). Analgesic properties of enkephalinase inhibitors: animal and human studies. *Prog. Clin. Biol. Res.*, **192**, 363–370.

Ernst, M. and Lee, M. H. M. (1987). Influence of naloxone on electro-acupuncture analgesia using an experimental dental pain test. Review of possible mechanisms of action. *Acupunct. Electrother. Res.*, **12**, 5–22.

Gracely, R. H. (1991). Experimental pain models. In *Advances in Pain Research and Therapy* (M. Max, R. Portenoy, E. Laska, eds), pp. 33–47. New York: Raven.

Guo, H.-F., Tian, J., Wang, X., Fang, Y. *et al.* (1996). Brain substrates activated by electroacupuncture of different frequencies (1): comparative study on the expression of oncogene c-fos and genes coding for three opioid peptides. *Mol. Brain Res.*, **43**, 157–166.

Han, J-S. (1997). Physiology of acupuncture: review of thirty years of research. *J. Alt. Comp. Med.*, **3**(suppl. 1), S101–108.

Han, J. and Terenius, L. (1982). Neurochemical basis of acupuncture analgesia. *Annu. Rev. Pharmacol. Toxicol.*, **22**, 192–220.

Han, J. S., Xie, G. X., Shou, Z. F. *et al.* (1982). Enkephalin and beta-endorphin as mediators of electro-acupuncture analgesia in rabbits: an antiserum microinjection study. In Regulatory Peptides from Molecular Biology to Function (E. Costa & M. Trabucchi, ed.), pp. 369–377. New York: Raven Press.

Han, J. S., Xie, G. X., Ding, X. Z. and Fan, S. G. (1984). High and low frequency electroacupuncture analgesia are mediated by different opioid peptides. *Pain*, (suppl. 2), S369.

Han, J. S., Ding, X. Z. and Fan, S. G. (1986a). Cholecystokinin octapeptide (CCK-8): antagonism to electroacupuncture analgesia and a possible role in electroacupuncture tolerance. *Pain*, **27,** 101–115.

Han, J. S., Yu, L. C. and Shi, Y. S. (1986b). A mesolimbic loop of analgesia III. A neuronal pathway from nucleus accumbens to periaqeductal grey. *Asia Pacific J. Pharmacol.*, **1,** 17–22.

Han, J. S., Chen, X. H., Sun, S. L. *et al.* (1991). Effect of low- and high-frequency TENS on Met-enkephalin-Arg-Phe and dynorphin A immunoreactivity in human lumbar CSF. *Pain*, **47,** 259–298.

Hawkes, C. H. (1992). Endorphins: the basis of pleasure? *J. Neurol. Neurosurg. Psychiatry*, **55,** 247–250.

Hughes, J., Smith, T. W., Kosterlitz, H. W. *et al.* (1975). Identification of two related pentapeptides from the brain with potent opiate agonist activity. *Nature*, **258,** 577–579.

Ishimaru, K., Kawakita, K. and Sakita, M. (1995). Analgesic effects induced by TENS and electroacupuncture with different types of stimulating electrodes on deep tissues in human subjects. *Pain*, **63,** 181–187.

Johnson, M. I., Kundu, S., Ashton, C. H. *et al.* (1996). The analgesic effects of acupuncture on experimental pain threshold and somatosensory evoked potentials in healthy volunteers. *Comp. Ther. Med.*, **4,** 219–225.

Jones, A. K. P., Brown, W. D., Friston, K. J. *et al.* (1991). Cortical and subcortical localisation of response to pain in man using positron emission tomography. *Proc. R. Soc. Lond. B*, **244,** 39–44.

Kawakita, K. and Gotoh, K. (1996). Role of polymodal receptors in the acupuncture-mediated endogenous pain inhibiotory systems. *Prog. Brain Res.*, **113**, 507–523.

Knox, V. J., Shum, K. and McLaughlin, D. M. (1978). Hypnotic analgesia vs hypnotic analgesia in high and low hypnotically susceptible subjects. In *Hypnosis and its Bicentennial* (F. H. Frankel and H. S. Zamansky, eds), pp. 101–108. New York: Plenum.

Knox, V. J., Handfield-Jones, C. E. and Shum, K. (1979). Subject expectancy and the reduction of cold pressor pain with acupuncture and placebo acupuncture. *Psychosom. Med.*, **41,** 477–486.

Le Bars, D. and Willer, J. C. (1988). Letter. *Pain*, **32,** 259–260.

Lee, J-H. and Beitz, A. J. (1993). The distribution of brain-stem and spinal cord nuclei associated with different frequencies of electroacupuncture analgesia. *Pain*, **52,** 11–28.

Le Bars, D., Dickenson, A. H., Besson, J-M. (1979). Diffuse noxious inhibitory controls (DNIC). 1. Effects on dorsal horn convergent neurones in the rat. *Pain*, **6,** 283–304.

Li, C. L., Ahlberg, C. L. L. D., Lansdell, H. *et al.* (1975). Acupuncture and hypnosis: effects on induced pain. *Exp. Neurol.*, **49,** 272–280.

Litscher, G., Schwarz, G., Sandner-Kiesling, A. and Hadoldt, I. (1997). Transkranielle Doppler-Sonographie-Roboteergesteuerte Sonden zur Quantifizierung des Einflusses der Akupunktur. *Sonderdruck Biomed. Technik*, **42,** S116–S122.

Liu, X., Zhu, B. and Zhang, S-X. (1986). Relationship between electroacupuncture analgesia and descending pain inhibitory mechanism of nucleus raphe magnus. *Pain*, **24,** 383–396.

Liu, X., Jiang, M.-C., Huang, P.-B. and Zou, T. (1992). The role of afferent C fibers in electro-acupuncture of Zusanli point activating nucleus raphe magnus. *Chin. J. Physiol. Sci.*, **8,** 257–267.

Liu, Y. K., Varela, M. and Oswald, R. (1975). The correspondence between some motor points and acupuncture loci. *Am. J. Chin. Med.*, **3,** 347–358.

Lu, G-W. (1983). Characteristics of afferent fiber innervation on acupuncture points zusanli. *Am. J. Physiol.*, **245,** R606–R612.

Lundeberg, T. (1984). A comparative study of the pain alleviating effect of vibratory stimulation, transcutaneous electrical nerve stimulation, electroacupuncture and placebo. *Am. J. Chin. Med.*, **12,** 72–79.

Lundeberg, T., Laurell, G. and Thomas, M. (1988). Effect of acupuncture on sinus pain and experimentally induced pain. *Ear Nose Throat J.*, **67,** 565–575.

Lundeberg, T., Eriksson, S., Lundeberg, S. and Thomas, M. (1989). Acupuncture and sensory thresholds. *Am. J. Chin. Med.*, **17,** 99–110.

Lundeberg, T., Eriksson, S. V., Lundeberg, S. and Thomas, M. (1991). Effect of acupuncture and naloxone in patients with osteoarthritis pain. A sham acupuncture controlled study. *Pain Clin.*, **4,** 155–161.

Mann, F. (1992). *Reinventing Acupuncture.* Oxford: Butterworth-Heinemann.

Mayer, D. J. and Price, D. D. (1981). Letter. *Pain*, **11,** 273–275.

Mayer, D. J., Price, D. D. and Rafii, A. (1977). Antagonism of acupuncture analgesia in man by the narcotic antagonist naloxone. *Brain Res.*, **121,** 368–372.

Melzack, R. and Wall, P. D. (1965). Pain mechanisms: a new theory. *Science*, **150,** 971–979.

Melzack, R. and Wall, P. (1973). *The Challenge of Pain.* Harmondsworth: Penguin.

Melzack, R., Stillwell, D. M. and Fox, E. J. (1977). Trigger points and acupuncture points for pain: correlations and implications. *Pain*, **3,** 3–23.

Molsberger, A. and Hille, E. (1994). The analgesic effect of acupuncture in chronic tennis elbow pain. *Br. J. Rheumatol.*, **33,** 1162–1165.

Moret, V., Forster, A., Laverriere, M-C. *et al.* (1991). Mechanism of analgesia induced by hypnosis and acupuncture: is there a difference? *Pain*, **45,** 135–140.

Myers, S. J., Kama, M. N., Pai, L. T. and Clark, W. C. (1982). A model of clinical pain. Technique for evaluation of analgesic agents *Am. J. Phys. Med.*, **61,** 1–10.

Nappi, G., Facchinetti, F., Legnante, G. (1982). Different releasing effects of traditional manual acupuncture and electroacupuncture on proopiocortin-related peptides. *Acupunct. Electrother. Res.*, **7,** 93–103.

Oyama, T., Jin, T. and Yamaya, R. (1980). Profound analgesic effects of beta-endorphin in man. *Lancet*, **315,** 122–124.

Pauser, von G., Reichmann, C., Baum, M. *et al.* (1975). Beeinflussung der Schmerzempfindung, des Schmerzgefuehls und der vegetativen Lage des Organismus unter Akupunktur-'Analgesie'. *Wien. Klin. Wochenschr.*, **87,** 25–28 (in German).

Peking Acupuncture Anaesthesia Co-ordinating Group (1973). Preliminary study on the mechanism of acupuncture anaesthesia. *Sci. Sin.*, **16,** 447–456.

Pomeranz, B. and Cheng, R. (1979). Suppression of noxious responses in single neurons of cat spinal cord by electroacupuncture and its reversal by the opiate antagonist naloxone. *Exp. Neurol.*, **64,** 327–341.

Pomeranz, B., Cheng, R. and Law, P. (1977). Acupuncture reduces electrophysiological and behavioural responses to noxious stimuli: pituitary is implicated. *Exp. Neurol.*, **54,** 172–178.

Price, D. D., Rafii, A., Watkins, L. R. and Buckingham, B. (1984). A psychophysical analysis of acupuncture analgesia. *Pain*, **19,** 27–42.

Research Group of Acupuncture Anaesthesia, Peking Medical College (1974). The role of some neurotransmitters of brain in finger-acupuncture analgesia. *Sci. Sin.*, **17,** 112–130.

Saletu, B., Saletu, M., Brown, M. *et al.* (1975). Hypno-analgesia and acupuncture analgesia: a neurophysiological reality? *Neuropsychobiology*, **1,** 218–242.

Sandkuehler, J. (1996). The organization and function of endogenous antinociceptive systems. *Progress in Neurobiology*, **50,** 49– 81.

Shen, E., Ma, W-H. and Lan, C. (1978). Involvement of descending inhibition in the effect of acupuncture on the splanchnically evoked potential in the orbital cortex of cat. *Sci. Sin.*, **21,** 677–685.

Sjolund, B., Terenius, L. and Eriksson, M. (1977). Increased cerebrospinal fluid levels of endorphins after electro-acupuncture. *Acta Physiol. Scand.*, **100,** 382–384.

Sjolund, B. H. and Eriksson, M. B. E. (1979). The influence of naloxone on analgesia produced by peripheral conditioning stimulation. *Brain Res.*, **173,** 295–301.

Smith, G. M., Chiang, H. T., Kitz, R. J. and Antoon, A. (1974). Acupuncture and experimentally induced ischaemic pain. *Adv. Neurol.*, **4,** 827–832.

Soper, W. Y. and Melzack, R. (1982). Stimulation-produced analgesia: evidence for somatotopic organization in the midbrain. *Brain Res.*, **251,** 301–311.

Stacher, G., Wancura, I., Bauer, P. *et al.* (1975). Effect of acupuncture on pain threshold and pain tolerance determined by electrical stimulation of the skin: a controlled study. *Am. J. Chin. Med.*, **3,** 143–149.

Stern, J. A., Brown, M., Ulett, A. and Sletten, I. (1977). A comparison of hypnosis, acupuncture, morphine, valium, aspirin, and placebo in the management of experimentally induced pain. *Ann. N.Y. Acad. Sci.*, **296,** 175–183.

Stewart, D. J., Thomson, J. and Oswald, I. (1977). Acupuncture analgesia: an experimental investigation. *Br. Med. J.*, **1,** 67–70.

Takeda, W. and Wessel, J. (1994). Acupuncture for the treatment of pain of osteoarthritic knees. *Arthitis Care Res.*, 7, 118–122.

Takeshige, C., Sato, T., Mera, T. *et al.* (1992). Descending pain inhibitory system involved in acupuncture analgesia. *Brain. Res. Bull.*, **29,** 617–634.

Takeshige, C., Oka, K., Mizuno, T. *et al.* (1993). The acupuncture point and its connecting central pathway for producing acupuncture analgesia. *Brain. Res. Bull.*, **30,** 53–67.

Tang, N-M., Dong, H-W., Wang, X-M. *et al.* (1997). Cholecystokinin antisense RNA increases the analgesic effect induced by electroacupuncture or low dose morphine: conversion of low responder rats into high responders. *Pain*, **71,** 71–80.

Thomas, M., Eriksson, S. V. and Lundeberg, T. (1991). A comparative study of diazepam and acupuncture in patients with osteoarthritis. *Am. J. Chin. Med.*, **19,** 95–100.

Toda, K. and Ichioka, M. (1978). Electroacupuncture: relations between forelimb afferent impulses and suppression of jaw-opening reflex in the rat. *Exp. Neurol.*, **61,** 465–470.

Travell, J. G. and Simons, D. G. (1983). *Myofascial Pain and Dysfunction. The Trigger Point Manual.* Baltimore: Williams and Wilkins.

Umlauf, R. (1976). Acupuncture effect on experimental pain in humans. *Cas. Lek. Cesk.*, **115,** 852–855 (in Czech).

Uvnas-Moberg, K., Bruzelius, G., Alster, P. and Lundeberg, T. (1993). The antinociceptive effect of non-noxious sensory stimulation is mediated partly through oxytocinergic mechanisms. *Acta Physiol. Scand.*, **149,** 199–204.

Vickers, A. J. (1996). Can acupuncture have specific effects on health? A systematic review of acupuncture antiemesis trials. *J. R. Soc. Med.*, **89,** 303–311.

Vierck, C. J., Lineberry, C. G., Lee, P. K. and Calderwood, H. W. (1974). Prolonged hypalgesia following acupuncture in monkeys. *Life Sci.*, **15,** 1277–1289.

Vincent, C. A., Richardson, P. H., Black, J. J. and Pither, C. E. (1989). The significance of needle placement site in acupuncture. *J. Psychosom. Res.*, **33,** 489–496.

Wang, K., Yao, S., Xian, Y. and Hou, Z. (1985). A study of the receptive field of acupoints and the relationship between the characteristics of needling sensation and groups of afferent fibres. *Sci. Sin.*, **28,** 963–971.

Wang, Q., Mao, L-M. and Han, J-S. (1990). The role of periaqueductal gray in mediation of analgesia produced by different frequencies of electroacupuncture stimulation in rats. *Int. J. Neurosci.*, **53,** 167–172.

Woolf, C. J. (1979). Transcutaneous electrical nerve stimulation and the reaction to experimental pain in human subjects. *Pain*, **7,** 115–127.

Woolf, C. J. and Thompson, J. W. (1994). Stimulation-induced analgesia: transcutaneous electrical nerve stimulation (TENS) and vibration. In *Textbook of Pain* (P. D. Wall and R. Melzack, eds), pp. 1191–1208. Edinburgh: Churchill Livingstone.

Wu, C-C., Chen, M-F. and Lin, C-C. (1994). Absorption of subcutaneous injection of Tc-99m pertechnate via acupuncture points and non-acupuncture points. *Am. J. Chin. Med.*, **22,** 111–118.

Young, R. F. and Chambi, V. I. (1987). Pain relief by electrical stimulation of the periaqueductal and periventricular gray matter. *J. Neurosurg.*, **66,** 364–371.

Zhang, A., Xiaoping, P., Shaofen, X. *et al.* (1980). Endorphins and acupuncture analgesia. *Chin. Med. J.*, **93,** 673–680.

Zhao, F. Y., Meng, X. Z., Yu, S. D. *et al.* (1978). The effect of clomipramine and pargyline on finger pressing anesthesia for removal of impacted third molar. *J. Beijing Med. Coll.*, **2,** 79–82 (in Chinese).

4

Effects of sensory stimulation (acupuncture) on circulatory and immune systems

Thomas Lundeberg

Acupuncture is a treatment modality included in traditional Chinese medicine (TCM). The theoretical basis of TCM is not acceptable from a biological viewpoint and therefore acupuncture is looked upon with scepticism by the western medical society. An important reason for this scepticism is the general lack of scientific documentation. In recent years studies have appeared dealing with the effects of acupuncture in cardiovascular and immune disorders. The underlying mechanisms are often described and discussed in relation to TCM. Surprisingly, no penetrating discussions have dealt with the physiological background. It should be recognized that any effect of acupuncture must rest on physiological and psychological mechanisms. The effects of acupuncture must be through artificial activation of systems that have biological effects in functional situations (Bucinskaite *et al.*, 1994, 1996, 1998; Andersson and Lundeberg, 1995; Wyon *et al.*, 1995, 1998).

In acupuncture, many different mechanisms are involved and similar results may be obtained with other types of mechanical, thermal and electrical stimulation and physical exercise. Acupuncture or needle stimulation results in the activation of high-threshold mechanical receptors in the stimulated tissue. In the skeletal muscle these receptors are innervated by A-delta fibres and C fibres. These receptors are physiologically activated by strong muscle contractions and have been denoted ergoreceptors. Functionally these receptors are excited during intense physical exercise, and therefore it may be suggested that the therapeutic effects attributed to acupuncture can also be noted during physical exercise and vice versa. This is supported by studies showing that both acupuncture and exercise results in the release of endogenous opioids such as beta-endorphin. Other kinds of high-threshold mechanoreceptors also being activated during acupuncture are the nociceptors.

Stimulation of ergo- and nociceptors results in the activation of spinal and central reflex mechanisms and involves activation of the beta-endorphinergic system projecting from the hypothalamus to the periaqueductal grey in the brainstem.

It is likely that acupuncture, through activation of the beta-endorphinergic system, affects vasomotor areas in the brainstem, thereby regulating the sympathetic tone. The sympathetic effects of sensory stimulation as well as muscle exercise can be separated into two phases:

excitation and depression. During the first phase there is an increased sympathetic tone with increased heart rate, blood pressure and cardiac output. Provided that the sensory stimulation continues for a sufficient period of time (about 20–40 minutes), endogenous opioids are released, which produce central inhibition of the autonomic outflow (post-stimulatory sympathetic inhibition). This sympathetic inhibition is not evident during the stimulation owing to excitatory input via somatic afferents and metabolic effects on chemoreceptors and is dependent on the functional state of the body. Thus, acupuncture decreases the sympathetic activity in hypertension (resulting in a decreased blood pressure) but gives the opposite effects in the hypotensive state (resulting in an increased blood pressure). This is probably related to the regulatory function of the baroreceptor reflex and different sensitivity of baroreceptors in hypo- and hypertension. It is possible that these regulatory mechanisms are part of a homoeostatic response. In studies on volunteers, Ballegaard and collaborators (1993) demonstrated that acupuncture reduced skin temperatures that were initially high, raised those that were low and had little effect on intermediate temperatures. In addition, they observed that changes in pulse and blood pressure (BP) were also regulated towards normal. The majority of work concerning sensory stimulation on cardiovascular responses highlights the importance of sympathetic, not vagal, nerves as the efferent reflex limb. This conclusion sometimes contradicts the findings in conscious humans where the contribution of the vagus nerve to the reflex arc should be borne in mind (Nishijo *et al.*, 1991). This is supported by our preliminary findings, in patients with borderline hypertension, showing increased vagal (parasympathetic) activity after acupuncture stimulation.

Via another system, beta-endorphin and other hormones are released to the blood (Uvnäs-Moberg *et al.*, 1993; Andersson and Lundeberg 1995). Proopiomelanocortin in the hypothalamus produces beta-endorphin, adrenocorticotrophic hormone (ACTH) and melanocyte stimulating hormone (MSH) following sensory stimulation. These hormones reach different target organs and play important roles in stress and immune responses. It is important to emphasize that the two beta-endorphinergic systems probably operate independently but that both may be activated during sensory stimulation.

Circulatory effects

The cardiovascular system was first observed to be under the influence of neural, humoral and local metabolic factors in 1847 when Carl Ludwig developed a method of continuously recording arterial blood pressure. Neural regulation was found to depend on mental or emotional and somatosensory influences, and on baroreceptor and chemoreceptor influences.

Effects of sensory stimulation (acupuncture) on peripheral blood flow

Patients are known to often remark on a feeling of warmth during acupuncture. Experimental evidence for peripheral effects of acupuncture and other modes of sensory stimulation has been provided by Lundeberg (1993) and Blom and collaborators (1993b). In one study, 21 patients with severe xerostomia were randomized to receive either acupuncture (11) or placebo needling (10). Those who received acupuncture showed increased salivary flow during and after the treatment, with improvement persisting throughout the observation year. Those who received placebo showed some improvement only during the actual treatment. A subsequent study aimed at investigating the influence of different modes of sensory stimulation on Sjögren's syndrome by comparing the effects of manual stimulation, low-frequency (2 Hz) electroacupuncture (EA), high frequency (80 Hz) EA and superficial needling as controls. The effects of acupuncture were assessed by blood flux ('flow'), which was measured from 20 minutes before the commencement of treatment until 20 minutes after the removal of the acupuncture needles. Significant changes in blood flux were seen both during and after manual stimulation and low-frequency acupuncture, compared with the controls. Patients who showed a more pronounced increase in blood flux during the different modes of acupuncture also reacted with increased salivary flow.

Ernst and Lee (1986), using thermography, found electroacupuncture produced a temporary increase in sympathetic tone locally during stimulation and, following stimulation, a sustained decrease in sympathetic tone as shown by vasodilatation could be recorded throughout the body, especially in the hands. To assess the effects of acupuncture in Raynaud's syndrome, Moehrle and colleagues (1995) conducted a randomized controlled trial using genuine or sham stimulation on subjects suffering from primary and secondary Raynaud's. Blood flow during cold stress was gauged by red cell velocity, measured with Doppler flowmeter and capillaroscopy. Primary Raynaud's subjects who received active treatment showed a significant reduction in the rate of attacks and increase in blood flow, while those with secondary symptoms displayed only a trend towards positive effects. No significant changes were seen in any of those receiving sham treatment.

In experimental studies evaluating the effects of different modes of sensory stimulation in ischaemic flaps in rats, increased blood flux and flap survival were obtained (Jansen *et al.*, 1989b). The results suggested that sensory nerve stimulation might be of clinical use in reconstructive surgery. This is supported by a clinical study using transcutaneous electrical nerve stimulation (TENS) to reverse ischaemia in 24 patients undergoing reconstructive surgery for mammary carcinoma. In 12 out of 14 patients in the treatment group, repeated TENS restored capillary filling to normal and reduced oedema and stasis. Only two out of the ten patients in the control group given placebo-TENS for 7 days showed any improvement with capillary refilling returning to normal (Lundeberg *et al.*, 1988).

Low-frequency TENS (2 Hz TENS) was also seen to produce vasodilatation in patients with diabetic polyneuropathy (Kaada, 1982), with a rise in skin temperature after about 20 minutes' application and lasting for 4–6 hours. The vasodilatation was found not to be reversible by naloxone, atropine, propanolol or other chemical blockades, and it was suggested that the effect was due to a release of the vasodilatory neuropeptide vasoactive intestinal polypeptide (VIP) involved in the mechanism. Also, high-frequency TENS (80 Hz TENS) has been shown to increase capillary blood flow in surgical flaps (Lundeberg *et al.*, 1988) in a manner which is very similar to the response to calcitonin gene-related peptide (CGRP).

Taken together the results suggest that acupuncture may affect the peripheral blood flow and that this effect may be explained by both peripheral and central effects.

Effects of acupuncture on blood pressure

As early as 1895, Hunt, in animal experiments, observed that weak stimuli to the central cut end of a somatic nerve caused depressor responses in arterial blood pressure, while higher stimulus strengths brought about pressor effects. He suggested that the peripheral nerves contained two types of afferents, characterized by differences in sensitivity to electrical stimuli. Laporte and Montastruc (1957) reported on the effectiveness of the various types of somatic afferents, classified by fibre diameter, and Johansson (1962) in more detail found that repetitive stimulation of myelinated cutaneous afferents produced depressor responses that were probably due to the activation of group III afferents. Stimulus intensities sufficient to excite group IV afferents resulted in pressor responses, irrespective of the impulse frequencies used.

Coote *et al.* (1971) and McCloskey and Mitchell (1972) observed that in anaesthetized animals tetanic contraction of the hindlimbs elicited by stimulation of the spinal nerves caused a rise in arterial blood pressure, usually with small increases in heart rate and pulmonary ventilation, suggesting the existence of metabolic (chemo-) receptors in skeletal muscles. Yao and collaborators (1982a,b) used acupuncture-like stimulation in spontaneously hypertensive rats (SHR) and compared it with the effects obtained in normotensive rats. There was an initial rise in blood pressure in both groups, followed by a prolonged fall that was much more marked in the hypertensive group. A reduction in sympathetic tone was observed by measuring the rate of firing in the splanchnic nerve, an effect that was seen to be reversed both by naloxone and the reduction of serotonin production. It is important to remember that the state of the experimental animal also affects the outcome and that some of the effects are only seen in conscious animals (Kline *et al.*, 1978; Li *et al.*, 1983). It has been suggested that the human equivalent of the spontaneous hypertensive rats studied by Yao and collaborators (1982a,b) are patients suffering from essential hypertension. Interestingly, a decrease in blood pressure has been reported in acupuncture-treated patients with essential hypertension (Rutkowsky, 1980; Tam and Yiu, 1975). In most patients the decrease in diastolic pressure was 5–10 mmHg. This would suggest that acupuncture may serve as an adjunct to conventional therapy and not as a sole treatment. Also, auricular acupuncture has been reported to reduce the blood pressure in the short term (Gaponjuk *et al.*, 1993).

The effect of acupuncture on blood pressure appears to be related both to the mode of stimulation and to the cause of hypertension. Most studies suggest that acupuncture may reduce hypertension at least in the short term, and this is encouraging for further investigation.

Effects of acupuncture in angina

Angina is considered to respond well to placebo and therefore sham-controlled studies are crucial in its research. However, several uncontrolled studies suggest acupuncture may have good effects in the treatment of angina. In 1991 Richter and co-workers compared individualized acupuncture with placebo tablet treatment in a crossover trial with 21 patients. The average number of anginal attacks fell from 12 per 4 weeks in the run-in period to 10.6 with the tablets, and to only 6.1 in the acupuncture period. Ballegaard and associates (1990) randomized stable angina patients to acupuncture treatment sessions, one group being needled at recognized points, the other at so-called 'non-acupuncture' points, but within the same segments. There was little difference between the groups in each study, although those of the second group had a better response in the form of a reduction in glyceryl nitrate consumption and angina attack rate. Their angina was relatively less severe than of those in the first study. From these results it was concluded that the effects of both treatments were non-specific (placebo), or that both interventions have a genuine effect which is not point specific. In a follow-up study, Ballegaard and colleagues (1991) studied the skin temperature changes in response to electroacupuncture in a portion of the original patients, and found that those whose angina had been helped were significantly more likely to show a rise in skin temperature with acupuncture. In 1995 they also reported positive effects on exercise tolerance, cardiac work capacity and a decreased glyceryl nitrate consumption, while expectation, personality and psychosocial factors did not correlate to the outcome (Ballegaard *et al.*, 1995). The hypothesis that acupuncture reduces sympathetic tone derives support from these studies, although it is possible that a vasodilator may be released by acupuncture or that pain may be relieved by acupuncture which in turn leads to reduced sympathetic tone. It should also be stressed that it is possible that all the above effects may be attributed to non-specific effects.

It may be concluded that acupuncture's ability to relieve pain could be of value in the management of angina. Acupuncture should be used to support conventional medical management and not as a substitute for it.

Acupuncture and the immune system

In the 1930s, experiments in conscious rats demonstrated that various harmful or stressful stimuli produced haemorrhage of the gastric mucosa, hypertrophy of the adrenal glands and atrophy of the thymus, the last suggesting reduction in immune function. For many years, it was believed that suppression of the immune system was mediated by glucocorticoids; however, when it was shown that stress-induced immunosuppression occurs in adrenalectomized as well as normal rats, it became clear that other factors (including neuronal) must also be involved. Some immune organs such as the thymus, the lymph nodes and spleen are innervated by autonomic efferent nerves whose fibres have been demonstrated to influence blood flow and the immune function itself in these organs (Bulloch, 1987). Electrical stimulation of vagal efferent nerves increases the release of lymphocytes from the thymus, and the release is decreased if the vagal nerves are severed (Antonica *et al.*, 1994). Sakic and co-workers (1989) used either manual or electroacupuncture to various points on rats for 2 days before and 4 days after injection of sheep red cells, with controls receiving no treatment or sham stimulation. Only treatment at a segmentally related point produced significantly lighter spleens and heavier adrenal glands than the controls. Lundeberg and colleagues (1991) found that acupuncture stimulation enhanced immune responses in conscious mice. The contribution of the sympathetic nervous system was analysed by applying blockers of sympathetic neurotransmitters. Fujiwara and colleagues (1991) confirmed the nerve pathways involved by showing that the response to stimulation was prevented by cutting the sciatic nerve or pretreating with naloxone. Kimura and associates (1994) used anaesthetized animals to eliminate emotional factors and prove that somatic afferent stimulation produces a reflex effect on immune function, with autonomic nerves acting as the efferent pathway. Electrical stimulation of splenic sympathetic nerves was found to decrease the cytotoxic activity of the natural killer (NK) cells in the spleen. Taken together, the above mentioned studies clearly demonstrate that immune organ functions are crucially dependent on neuronal influence.

Health was seen by the Chinese as a balance of yin and yang, and acupuncture was believed to correct imbalances between them. So it is claimed possible for acupuncture to be used to stimulate immune mechanisms as in the treatment of AIDS (Chen *et al.*, 1992), and to suppress the immune system as in the management of rhinitis, asthma, eczema, etc. The immune system is highly complex, and specialist knowledge is required to interpret functional tests. Often experiments are on isolated parts of the system, and reviews so far are more enthusiastic than systematic. However, Bossy (1994) has pointed out correlations between a modern understanding of acupuncture and the concepts of it within TCM. Stressful events like bereavement and depression in humans are also thought to affect the activity of NK cells and T lymphocytes. Acupuncture appears to have the potential to modulate the immune system. It releases beta-endorphin from the hypothalamus, and modulates the sympathetic nervous system via the brainstem. At the same time non-specific effects of treatment, empathy within the doctor–patient relationship, the listening, touch and ensuing relaxation will themselves have effects on the immune system. A logical base for point selection based on the theory of endorphin release and autonomic activity suggests the use of points around the affected organ, those at the segmental level of the spleen, and general points most likely to have a strong effect on opioid release. Auricular points may also be useful resulting in increased vagal efferent activity. Moxibustion, the heating of needles in situ, is traditionally regularly prescribed and experimental studies indicate that it causes an inhibition of the sympathetic tone. However, intense moxibustion probably has opposite effects.

Patients suffering from severe chronic bronchitis who had been taking either oral or injectable corticosteroids for many years and showed resulting leukocyte migration impairment, were given acupuncture at various chest and back points (Sliwinski and Kulej, 1989). Steroids were stopped at the start of the trial, although they had to be reintroduced briefly for some patients. Results showed that leukocyte migration turned towards normal in most patients during the course of 42 treatments, and it was concluded that further studies were warranted. Intensive moxibustion at the umbilicus was used by Ouyang and co-workers (1992) on 36 of 69 patients with lung cancer. The treatment group showed a significant increase in CD4 and CD11 cells compared with the untreated controls. Improvements were also seen in their digestion, respiration and mental attitudes. Warm needling was also studied by Liu *et al.* (1993) in treating rheumatoid arthritis. They found no significant changes in numbers of T lymphocytes, NK cells and levels of immunoglobulin after 30 treatments. Acupuncture used on patients with lung, oesophagus or stomach cancer (Xia *et al.*, 1986) produced less weight loss, increase in lymphocyte rosettes and general improvement of symptoms compared with controls. All patients had continued with their radio- or chemotherapy.

Several authors have reported on simple cell counts and immunoglobulin levels, but these have limited values. Acupuncture used as part of the anaesthetic process during major surgery did not protect the patients from the usual fall in white cell counts (Kho *et al.*, 1991) and it was felt treatments should be continued postoperatively to obtain effects on the immune system. A study by Zhou and collaborators (1988) tends to support this. Strong stimulation daily for 3 days after operation significantly increased phagocytic activity in patients compared with untreated controls.

Acute rhinitis is listed by the WHO for treatment by acupuncture, and it appears most responsive when the allergic component is the most prominent, as in hayfever. It is thought that local needling may produce immediate reflex vasoconstriction, reducing the symptoms of sneezing, blockage and irritation. Distal points may influence the immune system and thereby reduce the allergic response. Bu and Nakano (1990) measured the resistance to airflow through the nasal passages of 10 hayfever sufferers with a rhinomanometer. Different acupuncture points were used singly, and a local point was found to increase the nasal airflow by 50% in seven of the ten patients, supporting a local reflex action. In an uncontrolled clinical study Lau *et al.* (1975) found reductions in symptoms – congestion, sneezing, nasal discharge and itch – accompanied by significant reductions in eosinophil numbers and IgE levels in blood and nasal secretions in 22 patients with perennial rhinitis. However a recurrence of symptoms was seen in one-third of them at the 2-month follow-up, highlighting the importance of follow-ups in the interpretation of true clinical results. Following a pilot study where only one acupuncture point was stimulated and results favoured these patients over others receiving standard medication, Williamson and co-workers (1996) randomized 102 patients to either acupuncture (evoking DeQi) at three points including segmental and distal or to 'sham' acupuncture subcutaneously over the patella. There was no significant difference between the groups in assessing outcome, although during treatment 39% of the active treatment group reported remission of symptoms against 45% of the controls.

As yet no rigorous proof has been found to determine that the human immune system responds to needling in different ways under different conditions. However, studies do indicate that acupuncture might have a useful role in modifying immunological processes, and further clinical studies are justified. The effects of acupuncture may be attributed both to a general release of ACTH/cortisol and to segmental reflex mechanisms.

Acupuncture in dry mouth (xerostomia)

Xerostomia (dry mouth) is a well-known symptom of some systemic diseases, for example primary and secondary Sjögren's syndrome, as well as an unwanted side-effect of radiation treatment or medication. It may cause many problems for the affected patient, including difficulties in speaking, eating and swallowing, caries and infections of the oral mucosa, inability to wear dentures and altered sense of taste, and therefore it can be both physically and socially handicapping (Talal, 1987; Sreebny *et al.*, 1992). Different kinds of techniques have been developed in order to alleviate xerostomia; stimulation of salivary secretion by chewing gums or tablets, and saliva substitutes ranging between plain water and *ex tempore* concoctions that try to mimic natural saliva (Talal, 1987; Bjornstrom *et al.*, 1990). Medications such as pilocarpine and nicotinamide have been tried but with minor success (e.g. Schuller *et al.*, 1989). Also, battery-operated devices applied to the palate and tongue have been tried (e.g. Steller *et al.*, 1988). All these methods have one thing in common: their ameliorating effect lasts only for a short period of time. During the last decade patients with xerostomia of different aetiologies have been offered acupuncture. The results show that their salivary flow rates can be increased with this method and that the improvement often lasts for long periods (Blom *et al.*, 1992, 1993a, 1996).

To elucidate the effects of acupuncture, both animal and human studies have been carried out. It has been found that acupuncture stimulation affects both the central nervous system (CNS) and the autonomic nervous system (ANS) (see Chapter 3). However, it is also possible that the effects of acupuncture may be attributed to peripheral effects, by increasing the release of neuropeptides from peripheral nerve endings (PNS) (Kaada *et al.*, 1984; Jansen *et al.*, 1989a,b; Tsai *et al.*, 1989; Lundeberg *et al.*, 1991), resulting in similar effects to those seen following muscle exercise (Bucinskaite *et al.*, 1996; Lind *et al.*, 1996). One of the neuropeptides that is affected by sensory stimulation is calcitonin gene-related peptide (CGRP). This peptide consists of 37 amino acids, and it exerts a wide range of effects on gastrointestinal, endocrine, cardiovascular and tracheobronchial systems. CGRP is involved in neurogenic inflammatory reactions and modulates response to substance P (SP) in neurogenic inflammation; it causes endogenous vasodilatation and acts by releasing an endothelium-derived relaxing factor/nitrous oxide (EDRF/NO). CGRP does not cause extravasation but strongly potentiates the increase in extravasation produced by SP. It has a relaxant effect on vascular smooth muscle and can increase the blood flow in the skin, an effect that persists for several hours. CGRP coexists with SP in many primary afferents and monitors noxious events together with SP. It plays a part in pain perception; potentiates the hyperalgesia caused by SP and conveys nociceptive information to the first synapse in the spinal cord, where pain is processed (Kjartansson *et al.*, 1988; Jansen *et al.*, 1989a; Kerkut and Phillis, 1995). CGRP induces a delayed increase in salivary secretion (Ekstrom *et al.*, 1988) and its concentration in the saliva can be affected by pathology (Nicoladi and Del Banco, 1990).

The salivary secretion is controlled by the ANS. The parasympathetic system is dominant and it induces a powerful increase of the salivary secretion rates with low protein content. It causes contraction of myoepithelial cells and vasodilatation of capillaries in the salivary glands, which leads to increased blood flow. The sympathetic system has a more intermittent role; when activated it causes a low, viscous salivary flow (Garrett and Kidd, 1993). The salivary secretion is also affected by other transmitters apart from acetylcholine and norepinephrine, viz. neuropeptides, which can regulate the volume of the saliva produced by increasing the blood flow in the salivary glands and affecting the secretion itself (Hauser-Kronberger *et al.*, 1992; Herbst *et al.*, 1992).

In order to elucidate the mechanisms behind the effect of acupuncture on salivary secretion in xerostomia sufferers, Dawidson and collaborators have conducted several studies concerning the connection between salivary secretion, neuropeptides and acupuncture. They found that acupuncture stimulation increases the blood flux in the skin over the parotid gland in patients with Sjögren's syndrome (Blom *et al.*, 1993b). They also reported that the neuropeptide concentration in saliva varies with secretion rates (Dawidson *et al.*, 1997) and that the concentration of some neuropeptides can be increased in the saliva of healthy subjects with acupuncture stimulation (Dawidson *et al.*, 1998a). In a recent study it was found that the concentration of vasoactive intestinal polypeptide (VIP) increased after the acupuncture treatment, when compared with baseline levels, in the saliva of xerostomic patients (Dawidson *et al.*, 1998b).

In ongoing studies, Dawidson and colleagues have investigated the influence of acupuncture stimulation on the concentration of CGRP in the saliva of xerostomia sufferers. They hypothesized that acupuncture stimulation could increase the release of CGRP from the nerve endings of the autonomic and/or sensory nervous system, thus leading to an increase of salivary flow. Out of 65 patients who were treated with acupuncture for xerostomia, 17 were chosen to participate in that study due to their ability to produce enough stimulated saliva for the radioimmunoassay (RIA) analyses prior to the start of the study. They were able to conduct RIA analyses of CGRP on the saliva of 14 of these patients, six men and eight women, aged 37–71, median 56 years. The periods of time that they have suffered from xerostomia varied from a few months (after radiation treatment) to several years for the secondary Sjögren's patients. Using standardized salivary flow test procedures, they collected paraffin-chewing stimulated saliva from the patients before the beginning of the study and then after the acupuncture treatment was completed. The acupuncture treatment was performed by an experienced acupuncturist (M. Blom), using the same points as in earlier studies when xerostomia was treated with sensory stimulation (Blom *et al.*, 1992). The following points were used bilaterally: ST 3, ST 6 in the face, LI 4 in the hands and ST 36 and SP 6 in the legs. After standard disinfecting of the site, the needles were inserted through the skin to the depth of 5–10 mm, and manipulated until the needle sensation (DeQi) was elicited. When that sensation had been achieved, the needles were left *in situ* and not manipulated again unless a needle was displaced. All patients received two series of acupuncture treatments in 24 sessions of 20 minutes each. The results show that the concentrations of CGRP in the saliva of the patients were significantly higher after the end of acupuncture treatment as compared to the baseline levels before acupuncture ($P<0.001$). The increased release of the neuropeptide CGRP could be one of the factors that contribute to the salivary secretion.

Dawidson and collaborators have suggested that VIP can act as a trophic factor on the salivary gland tissues. It is possible that CGRP has a similar function apart from its influence on the salivary secretion rates. According to Dalsgaard *et al.* (1989), CGRP has trophic influence on the endothelial cells, and might positively affect the microcirculation in the capillary vessels. The salivary glands contain considerable amounts of growth factors, which exert a trophic effect on the neurones of the autonomic and sensory nervous system (Sporn *et al.*, 1983; Zelles *et al.*, 1995). Acupuncture stimulation may produce a release of the nerve growth factors (NGF) which affect the sensory and autonomic nervous systems, by inducing an increase in the production of CGRP and VIP in the nerve cells, and subsequent release of that CGRP and VIP in target organs, in this case the salivary glands. Such a course might be the explanation of the long-term effect of acupuncture treatment.

Conclusion

In the treatment of diseases with sensory stimulation the engagement of the patient is important. The contribution of psychological factors is crucial, especially when using methods activating endogenous systems. In elegant experimental studies evaluating the effects of sensory stimulation on pain thresholds, Andersson and collaborators (Widerström-Noga, 1993; Dyrehag 1998) have demonstrated that patients with high anxiety report no effect of acupuncture, whereas patients with low anxiety had increased pain thresholds.

To obtain an effect the somatic and psychological factors must act in harmony to utilize endogenous mechanisms most effectively. Also, the patient must be responsive to treatment (Thomas and Lundeberg, 1996).

References

Andersson S. and Lundeberg T. (1995). Acupuncture from empiricism to science: functional background to acupuncture effects in pain and disease. *Med. Hypotheses*, **45,** 271–281.

Antonica, A., Magni, F., Mearini, L. and Paolocci, N. (1994). Vagal control of lymphocyte release from rat thymus. *J. Auton. Nerv. Syst.*, **48,** 187–197.

Ballegaard, S., Pedersen, F., Pietersen, A. *et al.* (1990). Effects of acupuncture in moderate, stable angina pectoris: a controlled study. *J. Int. Med.*, **227,** 25–30.

Ballegaard, S., Meyer, C. N. and Trojaborg, W. (1991). Acupuncture in angina pectoris: does acupuncture have a specific effect? *J. Int. Med.*, **229,** 357–362.

Ballegaard, S., Muteki, T., Harada, H. *et al.* (1993). Modulatory effects of acupuncture on the cardiovascular system: a cross-over study. *Acupunct. Electrother. Res.*, **18,** 103–115.

Ballegaard, S., Karpatschoff, B., Holck, J. *et al.* (1995). Acupuncture in angina pectoris: do psycho-social and neurophysiological factors relate to the effect? *Acupunct. Electrother. Res.*, **20,** 101–116.

Bjornstrom, M., Axell, T. and Birkhed, D. (1990). Comparison between saliva stimulants and saliva substitutes in patients with symptoms related to dry mouth. *Swed Dent. J.*, **14,** 153–161.

Blom, M., Dawidson, I. and Angmar-Månsson, B. (1992). The effect of acupuncture on salivary flow rates in patients with xerostomia. *Oral Surg. Oral Med. Oral Pathol.*, **73,** 293–298.

Blom, M., Dawidson, I. and Angmar-Månsson, B. (1993a). Acupuncture treatment of xerostomia caused by irradiation treatment of the head and neck region – two case reports. *J. Oral Rehabil.*, **20,** 491–494.

Blom, M., Lundeberg, T., Dawidson, I. and Angmar-Månsson, B. (1993b). Effect of acupuncture on blood flow in patients suffering from xerostomia. *Oral Rehabil.*, **73,** 541–548.

Blom, M., Dawidson, I., Fernberg, J-O. *et al.* (1996). Acupuncture treatment of patients with radiation-induced xerostomia. *Oral Oncol. Eur. J. Cancer*, **32B,** 182–190.

Bossy, J. (1994). Acupuncture and immunity: basic and clinical aspects. *Acupunct. Med.*, **12,** 60–62.

Bu, G. and Nakano, T. (1990). Clinical application of rhinomanometer. *Chin. Med. J.*, **103,** 956–958.

Bucinskaite, V., Lundeberg, T., Stenfors, C. *et al.* (1994). Effects of electro-acupuncture and physical exercise on regional concentrations of neuropeptides in rat brain. *Brain Res.*, **666,** 128–132.

Bucinskaite, V., Theodorsson, E., Crumpton, K. *et al.* (1996). Effects of repeated sensory stimulation (electro-acupuncture) and physical exercise (running) on open-field behaviour and concentrations of neuropeptides in the hippocampus in WKY and SHR rats. *Eur. J. Neurosci.*, **8,** 382–387.

Bucinskaite, V., Crumpton, K., Theodorsson E. and Lundeberg T. (1998). Sensory stimulation (electro-acupuncture) and physical exercise effects on blood pressure and nociception. *Int. J. Neurosci.*, **34,** 1–12.

Bulloch, K. (1987). The innervation of immune system tissues and organs. In: *The Neuro–Immune–Endocrine Connection* (C. W. Cotman, R. E. Brinton, A. Galaburda *et al.*, eds), pp. 29–78. New York: Raven.

Chen, H., Cai, D., Zhai, D. and Zhao, C. (1992). Investigation on the flexibility of treating AIDS with acupuncture and moxibustion. *Int. J. Clin. Acupunct.*, **11,** 193–195.

Coote, J. H., Hilton, S. M. and Perez-Gonzalez, J. F. (1971). The reflex nature of the pressor response to muscular exercise. *J. Physiol. (Lond.)*, **215,** 789–804.

Dalsgaard, C-J., Hultgardh-Nilsson, A., Haegerstrand, A. and Nilsson, J. (1989). Neuropeptides as growth factors. Possible roles in human diseases. *Regul. Pept.*, **25,** 1–9.

Dawidson, I., Blom, M., Lundeberg, T. *et al.* (1997). Neuropeptides in the saliva of healthy subjects. *Life Sci.*, **60,** 269–278.

Dawidson, I., Angmar-Månsson, B., Blom, M. *et al.* (1998a). The influence of sensory stimulation (acupuncture) on the release of neuropeptides in the saliva of healthy subjects. *Life Sci.*, **63,** 659–674.

Dawidson, I., Angmar-Månsson, B., Blom, M. *et al.* (1998b). Sensory stimulation (acupuncture) increases the release of vasoactive intestinal polypeptide in the saliva of xerostomia sufferers. *Neuropeptides* , **32**,(6), 543–548.

Dyrehag, L-E. (1998). Effects of Somatic Afferent Stimulation in Chronic Musculoskeletal Pain. Thesis, University of Gothenburg, Sweden.

Ekström, J., Ekman, R., Håkanson, R. *et al.* (1988). Calcitonin gene-related peptide in rat salivary glands: neuronal localization, depletion upon nerve stimulation, and effects on salivation in relation to substance P. *Neuroscience*, **26,** 933–949.

Ernst, M. and Lee, M. H. M. (1986). Sympathetic effects of manual and electrical acupuncture of the Tsuanli knee point: comparison with the Hoku hand point sympathetic effect. *Exp. Neurol.*, **94,** 1–10.

Fujiwara, R., Zhou, G. T., Matsuoka, H. *et al.* (1991). Effects of acupuncture on immune response in mice. *Int. J. Neurosci.*, **57,** 141–150.

Gaponjuk, P. J., Shekovina, T. J. and Leonova, M. V. (1993). Clinical effectiveness of auricular acupuncture treatment of patients with hypertensive disease. *Acupunct. Med.*, **11,** 29–31.

Garrett, J. R. and Kidd, A. (1993). The innervation of salivary glands as revealed by morphological methods. *Microsc. Res. Tech.* **26,** 75–91.

Hauser-Kronberger, C., Albegger, K., Saria, A. and Hacker G. W. (1992). Neuropeptides in human salivary (submandibular and parotid) glands. *Acta Otolaryngol. (Stockh).*, **112,** 343–348.

Herbst, W. M., Kummer, W. and Heym, C. (1992). Localization of vasoactive intestinal polypeptide-receptor-immunoreactivity in human salivary glands. *Neuropeptides*, **22,** 89–92.

Hunt, R. (1895). The fall of blood pressure resulting from the stimulation of afferent nerves. *J. Physiol. (Lond.)*, **18,** 381–410.

Jansen, G., Lundeberg, T., Kjartansson, J. and Samuelson, U. E. (1989a). Acupuncture and sensory neuropeptides increase cutaneous blood flow in rats. *Neurosci. Lett.*, **97,** 305–309.

Jansen, G., Lundeberg, T., Samuelson, U. E. and Thomas, M. (1989b). Increased survival of ischaemic musculocutaneous flaps in rats after acupuncture. *Acta Physiol. Scand.*, **135,** 555–558.

Johansson, B. (1962). Circulatory responses to stimulation of somatic afferents. *Acta Physiol. Scand.*, **57**(suppl 198), 1–91.

Kaada, B. (1982). Vasodilation induced by transcutaneous nerve stimulation in peripheral ischaemia (Raynaud's phenomenon and diabetic polyneuropathy). *Eur. Heart J.*, **3,** 303–314.

Kaada, B., Olsen, E. and Eielsen, O. (1984). In search of mediators of skin vasodilation induced by transcutaneous nerve stimulation: III. Increase in plasma VIP in normal subjects and in Raynaud's disease. *Gen. Pharmacol.*, **15,** 107–113.

Kerkut, A. and Phillis, J. W. (1995). Tachykinins and calcitonin gene-related peptide (CGRP) as co-transmitters released from peripheral endings of sensory nerves. *Prog. Neurobiol.*, **45,** 1–98.

Kho, H. G., van Egmond, J., Eijk, R. J. R. and Kapteyns, W. M. M. J. (1991). Lack of influence of acupuncture and transcutaneous stimulation on the immunoglobulin levels and leukocyte counts following upper-abdominal surgery. *Eur. J. Anaesth.*, **8,** 39–45.

Kimura, A., Nagai, N. and Sato, A. (1994). Somatic afferent regulation of cytotoxic activity of splenic natural killer cells in anesthetized rats. *Jpn. J. Physiol.*, **44,** 651–664.

Kjartansson, J., Lundeberg, T., Samuelson, U. E. *et al.* (1988). Calcitonin Gene-related Peptides (CGRP) and transcutaneous electrical stimulation (TENS) increase cutaneous blood flow in a musculocutaneous flap in the rat. *Acta Physiol. Scand.*, **134,** 89–94.

Kline, R. L., Yeung, K. Y. and Calaresu, F. R. (1978). Role of somatic nerves in the cardiovascular responses to stimulation of an acupuncture point in anesthetized rabbits. *Exp. Neurol.*, **61,** 561–570.

Laporte, Y. and Montastruc, P. (1957). Rôle des types différents de fibres afférentes dans les réflexes circulatoires généraux d'origine cutanée. *J. Physiol. (Paris)*, **49,** 1039–1049.

Lau, B. H. S., Wong, D. S. and Slater, J. M. (1975). Effect of acupuncture on allergic rhinitis: clinical and laboratory evaluations. *Am. J. Chin. Med.*, **3,** 263–270.

Li, P., Sun, F-Y. and Zhang, A-Z. (1983). The effect of acupuncture on blood pressure: the interrelation of sympathetic activity and endogenous opioid peptides. *Acupunct. Electrother. Res.*, **8,** 45–56.

Lind, H., Brudin, L., Lindholm, L. and Edvinsson, L. (1996). Different levels of sensory neuropeptides (calcitonin gene-related peptide and substance P) during and after exercise in man. *Clin. Physiol.*, **16,** 73–82.

Liu, X., Sun, L. and Xiao, J. I. (1993). Effect of acupuncture and point-function in rheumatoid arthritis. *J. Trad. Chin. Med.*, **13,** 174–178.

Ludwig, C. (1847). Beiträge zur Kenntnis des Einflusses der Respirationsbewegungen auf den Blutlauf im Aortensysteme. *Joh. Mullers Arch. Anat. Physiol. Wiss. Med.*, 242.

Lundeberg, T. (1993). Peripheral effects of sensory nerve stimulation (acupuncture) in inflammation and ischemia. *Scand. J. Rehabil. Med.*, **S29,** 61–86.

Lundeberg, T., Kjartansson, J. and Samuelson, U. (1988). Effect of electrical nerve stimulation on healing of ischaemic skin flaps. *Lancet*, **2,** 712–715.

Lundeberg, T., Eriksson, V. and Theodorsson, E. (1991). Neuroimmunomodulatory effects of acupuncture in mice. *Neurosci. Lett.*, **128,** 161–164.

McCloskey, D. I. and Mitchell, J. H. (1972). Reflex cardiovascular and respiratory responses originating in exercising muscle. *J. Physiol. (Lond.)*, **224,** 173–186.

Moehrle, M., Blum, A., Lorenz, F. *et al.* (1995). Proceedings of the 2nd Asian Congress for Microcirculation, Beijing, p. 10.

Nicolodi, M. and Del Bianco, E. (1990). Sensory neuropeptides (substance P, calcitonin gene-related peptide and vasoactive intestinal polypeptide) in human saliva: their pattern in migraine and cluster headache. *Cephalalgia*, **10,** 39–50.

Nishijo, K., Enpin, U., Yoshikawa, K. *et al.* (1991). The neural mechanism of the response in heart rate induced by acupuncture. In *New Trends in Autonomic Nervous System Research* (M. Yoshikawa *et al.*, eds), p. 594. Amsterdam: Elsevier.

Ouyang, Z. R., Fan, L. and Gong, Q. H. (1992). Comparison of the effect of stimulating the femoral nerve, artery and lymphatic vessels with acupuncture at Zsusanli on intestinal motility in rabbits. *Shanghai J. Acupunct.*, **4,** 14–16.

Richter, A., Herlitz, J. and Hjalmarsson, A. (1991). Effect of acupuncture in patients with angina pectoris. *Eur. Heart J.*, **12,** 175–178.

Rutkowsky, B. (1980). Electrical stimulation and essential hypertension. *Acupunct. Electrother. Res.*, **5,** 287–295.

Sakic, B., Kojic, L., Jankovic, B. D. and Skokljev, A. (1989). Electro-acupuncture modifies humoral immune response in the rat. *Acupunct. Electrother. Res.*, **14,** 115–120.

Schuller, D. E., Stevens, P., Clausen, K. P. *et al.* (1989). Treatment of radiation side effects with oral Pilocarpine. *J. Surg. Oncol.*, **42,** 272–276.

Sliwinski, J. and Kulej, M. (1989). Acupuncture induced immunoregulatory influence on the clinical state of patients suffering from chronic spastic bronchitis and undergoing long-term treatment with corticosteroids. *Acupunct. Electrother. Res.*, **14,** 227–234.

Sporn, M. B., Roberts, A. B., Shull, J. H. *et al.* (1983). Polypeptide transforming growth factors isolated from bovine sources and used for wound healing in vivo. *Science*, **219,** 1329–1331.

Sreebny, L. M., Banoczy, J., Baum, B. J. *et al.* (1992). Saliva: its role in health and disease. *Int. Dent. J.*, **42(**suppl. 2), 287–304.

Steller, M., Chou, L. and Daniels, T. E. (1988). Electrical stimulation of salivary flow in patients with Sjögren's Syndrome. *J. Dent. Res.*, **67,** 1334–1337.

Talal, N. (1987). Overview of Sjögren's syndrome. *J. Dent. Res.*, **66,** 672–674.

Tam, K-C. and Yiu, H-H. (1975). The effect of acupuncture on essential hypertension. *Am. J. Chin. Med.*, **3,** 369–375.

Thomas, M. and Lundeberg, T. (1996). Does acupuncture work? *Pain Clin. Updates*, **4,** 1–4.

Tsai, H. Y., Lin, J. G. and Inoki, R. (1989). Further evidence for possible analgesic mechanisms of electroacupuncture: effects on neuropeptides and serotonergic neurons in rat spinal cord. *Jpn. J. Pharmacol.*, **49,** 181–185.

Uvnäs-Moberg, K., Bruzelius, G., Alster, P. and Lundeberg, T. (1993). The antinociceptive effect of non-noxious sensory stimulation is mediated partly through oxytocinergic mechanisms. *Acta Physiol. Scand.*, **149,** 199–204.

Widerström-Noga, E. (1993). Analgesic Effects of Somatic Afferent Stimulation – A Psychobiological Perspective. Thesis, University of Gothenburg, Sweden.

Williamson, L., Yudkin, P., Livingstone, R. *et al.* (1996). Hay fever treatment in general practice: a randomised controlled trial comparing western acupuncture with sham acupuncture. *Acupunct. Med.*, **14,** 6–10.

Wyon, Y., Lindgren, R., Lundeberg, T. and Hammar, M. (1995). Effects of acupuncture on climacteric vasomotor symptoms, quality of life and urinary excretion of neuropeptides among postmenopausal women. *Menopause*, **2,** 3–12.

Wyon, Y., Hammar, M., Theodorsson, E. and Lundeberg T. (1998). Effects of physical activity and acupuncture on calcitonin gene-related peptide immunoreactivity in different parts of the rat brain and in cerebrospinal fluid, serum and urine. *Acta Physiol. Scand.*, **162,** 517–521.

Xia, Y. Q., Zhang, D., Yang, J. C. *et al.* (1986). An approach to the effect on tumours of acupuncture in combination with radiotherapy or chemotherapy. *J. Trad. Chin. Med.*, **6,** 23–26.

Yao, T., Andersson, S. and Thorén, P. (1982a). Long-lasting cardiovascular depression induced by acupuncture-like stimulation of the sciatic nerve in unanaesthetized spontaneously hypertensive rats. *Brain Res.*, **240,** 77–85.

Yao, T., Andersson, S. and Thorén, P. (1982b). Long-lasting cardiovascular depressor response following sciatic stimulation in SHR. Evidence for the involvement of central endorphin and serotonin systems. *Brain Res.*, **244,** 295–303.

Zelles, T., Purushotham, K. R., Macauley, S. P. *et al.* (1995). Saliva and growth factors: the fountain of youth resides in us all. *J. Dent. Res.*, **74,** 1826–1832.

Zhou, R., Huang, F., Jiang, S. and Jiang, J. (1988). The effect of acupuncture on the phagocytic activity of human leukocytes. *J Trad. Chin. Med.*, **8,** 83–84.

5

Clinical effectiveness of acupuncture: an overview of systematic reviews

Edzard Ernst

Introduction

In spite of its long history and (in the west) increasing prevalence, the clinical effectiveness of acupuncture has remained controversial. This is perhaps best borne out by the conclusions of a recent 'NIH Consensus Development Statement': 'There have been many studies of its potential usefulness. However, many of these studies provide equivocal results because of design, sample size, and other factors' (NIH, 1997).

Demonstrating the effectiveness of acupuncture is undoubtedly complex and notoriously complicated by a host of methodological issues (e.g. Vincent and Lewith, 1995; Ernst and White, 1997). During the last few years, this area has been evaluated by conducting a series of systematic reviews and meta-analyses. This chapter is aimed at summarizing this work. In particular, we ask whether acupuncture is effective as a treatment for the following conditions:

- Dental pain (Ernst and Pittler, 1998).
- Low back pain (Ernst and White, 1999).
- Neck pain (White and Ernst, 1999).
- Osteoarthritis (Ernst, 1997a).
- Stroke (Ernst and White, 1996).
- Smoking cessation (White *et al.*, 1999).
- Weight loss (Ernst, 1997b).

Work in relation to experimental pain is described in Chapter 3.

Full details of the methods of each separate piece of research are given in the respective publications (Ernst and White, 1996, 1999; Ernst, 1997a, b; Ernst and Pittler, 1998; White and Ernst, 1999; White *et al.*, 1999). A precise research question was formulated at the outset of each project. A thorough search for all published controlled clinical trials on each subject followed. Table 5.1 summarizes the various search strategies and other methodological details of each project. The papers for each review were chosen according to predefined inclusion/exclusion criteria. This was followed by standardized data extraction and (where possible) data synthesis.

Table 5.1 Summary of methodological details

Project/reference	*Acupuncture type*	*Databases searched*	*Main inclusion criteria*	*Main exclusion criteria*
dental pain (Ernst and Pittler, 1998)	any	Medline Embase CISCOM Cochrane library Own files	controlled trials on human volunteers/patients	trials comparing one form of acup. vs another
low back pain (Ernst and White, 1998)	needle only, with or without electrical stimulation	Medline CISCOM Cochrane library Own files	RCTs on human patients	trials comparing one form of acup. vs another Trials published in languages other than English, French, German, Spanish, Italian or Polish
neck pain (White and Ernst, 1999)	any	Medline, Embase Cochrane library CISCOM Own files	RCTs	headache only or pain in multiple sites Trials comparing one form of acup. vs another
osteoarthritis (Ernst, 1997a)	any	Medline CISCOM Own files	controlled trials on human patients	trials comparing one form of acup. vs another
stroke (Ernst and White, 1996)	any	Medline CISCOM Own files	controlled trials on human patients	trials comparing one form of acup. vs another
smoking cessation (White *et al.*, in press)	any	Medline Embase British Library CISCOM Science Citation Index Own files	sham-controlled, single-blind RCTs on smokers	trials published in languages other then English, French or German
weight loss (Ernst, 1997b)	any acup. or acupressure	Medline CISCOM Own files	randomized, sham-controlled trials	trials comparing one form of acup. vs another

Dental pain

A systematic review of acupuncture for dental pain included 16 controlled trials (Ernst and Pittler, 1998). The methodological quality of all trials was assessed by the Jadad score (Jadad *et al.*, 1996). With few exceptions, the trials were burdened with significant methodological flaws. Key data of all trials are summarized in Table 5.2.

Of the 16 studies, nine suggested that acupuncture had a significantly positive effect on either pain, pain threshold or pain-free time period after operation. Four trials had a negative result and three lacked formal test statistics. On the basis of this evidence, it was concluded that acupuncture can alleviate dental pain. Future investigations should overcome the methodological problems associated with some of the published studies, define the optimal acupuncture technique and evaluate its relative efficacy compared to conventional methods of analgesia used for dental pain.

Low back pain

A systematic review and meta-analysis was conducted on the subject of low back pain (Ernst and White, 1998). Again, the methodological quality of all trials was assessed by the Jadad score (Jadad *et al.*, 1996). In addition, the appropriateness of the acupuncture techniques was judged by a panel of experienced acupuncturists who were blinded to the origin of the publications (White and Ernst, 1998). Twelve studies met the inclusion/exclusion criteria (Table 5.1). Most related to chronic back pain. Key data of these trials are summarized in Table 5.3.

The majority of the trial results favoured acupuncture as an effective treatment of low back pain over various control interventions. The overall odds ratio of improvement with acupuncture compared to various control interventions, in the nine studies which presented data in suitable form, was 2.02 (95% CI 1.39–2.94). For trials which were both sham-controlled as well as patient and evaluator-blind, the result was not statistically significant. Interestingly, the effect of acupuncture was, if anything, slightly more pronounced for those trials which were judged by our expert panel to have employed inadequate acupuncture techniques. It was concluded that reasonably good evidence supports the use of acupuncture for low back pain. Unfortunately, numerous caveats prevent firmer conclusions.

Neck pain

A comprehensive search strategy was designed to retrieve all randomized controlled trials of acupuncture for neck pain. Twenty-four studies met our predefined inclusion and exclusion criteria (Table 5.1). The trials were highly heterogeneous and few were of acceptable quality as estimated by the Jadad score (Jadad *et al.*, 1996). The key data of all trials are summarized in Table 5.4.

Table 5.2 Controlled trials of acupuncture in dental pain

First author	*Reference*	*Design*	*No.*	*Interventions*	*Endpoint*	*Main result*
Bakke	*Scand. J. Dent. Res.* 1976; **84:**404–408	CCT	33 volunteers	A) without acup. B) manual acup. C) electroacup. D) TENS	pain threshold	significant increase of threshold with electroacup.
Brandwein	*Am. J. Acup.* 1976;**4:** 370–375	CCT	184 patients	A) lidocaine B) needle acup. (manual + electrical stimulation) C) lidocaine + acup.	pain during operation	in A, 70% felt no pain, in B 27% and in C 83% (no formal test statistics)
Chapman	*Pain* 1976;**2:**265–283	RCT observer- and patient-blind	60 healthy volunteers	A) needle acup. B) TENS at acup. point C) sham needle acup. D) no treatment	pain after painful dental stimuli	A and B showed a small but significant analgesic response
Chapman	*Pain* 1976;**3:**213–227	CCT	20 healthy volunteers	A) 80 min electroacup. at facial sites (2 Hz) B) no analgesic treatment	pain threshold	187% increase of pain threshold after acup.
Sung	*Anesth. Analg.* 1977;**56:** 473–478	RCT patient-blind, observer-blind	40 male patients	A) sham acup. + oral placebo B) sham acup. + 60 mg codeine C) acup. at 2 Hoku points + oral placebo D) acup. at 2 Hoku points + 60 mg codeine	pain intensity during 3 hours postoperatively	significant ($P<0.01$) pain relief in C vs A and in D vs B
Taub	*J. Am. Dent. Assoc.* 1977; **95:**555–561	RCT patient-blind	39 patients	A) trad acup. B) sham acup.	pain during operation (rated on 5-point scale by patient)	numerically less pain in A (no formal test statistics)

Taub	*Oral Surg. Oral Med. Oral Pathol.* 1979;**48:**205–210	RCT patient-blind, evaluator-blind	51 patients	electroacup. at Hoku points vs sham acup.	pain rated on a 5-point scale by patient and dentist	no intergroup differences. Success rate near 100% in both groups
Chapman	*Pain* 1982;**12:**319	CCT crossover	40 healthy volunteers	A) control session B) acup. session	pain after painful dental stimuli	decreased pain during the B sessions
Hansson	*Oral Surg.* 1987;**64:** 285–286	RCT	21 patients	preop formula acup.: A) = no stimulation B) = manual stimulation C) = electrical stimulation D) = electrical stimulation also during surgery	intraoperative pain by VAS + use of conventional analgesia	no intergroup differences reported. Only two patients tolerated extraction without conventional analgesia (and both reported severe pain)
Lapeer	*J. Can. Dent. Assoc.* 1987; **6:**479–480	RCT	18 patients	electroacup. vs conventional analgesics administered postoperatively	pain intensity + analgesic use	no intergroup differences
Kitade	*Int. J. Acup. Electrother. Res.* 1990;**15:**121–135	RCT patient-blind	56 patients	A) trad acup. + oral placebo vs B) trad acup + D-phenyl-alanine (B) (slows degradation of enkephalins)	pain during surgery rated by patient after tooth extraction on a 4-point scale	in group A there were good or excellent results in 42%, in group B 78%. No test statistics
Ekblom	*Pain* 1991;**44:**241–247	RCT	110 patients	A) preoperative acup. B) postoperative acup. C) no acup. (all received local anaesthetics)	pain during operation, pain after operation analgesics consumption	in A and B more pain after operation than C. In A more pain during operation and more analgesics consumption than C

Table 5.2 continued overleaf

Table 5.2 *continued*

First author	*Reference*	*Design*	*No.*	*Interventions*	*Endpoint*	*Main result*
Simmons	*Anesth. Prog.* 1993;**40:** 14–19	RCT double-blind, sham-controlled	40 volunteers	A) auricular electroacup. + saline i.v. B) auricular electroacup. + naloxone i.v. C) sham-auricular acup. + saline i.v. D) sham auricular acup. + naloxone i.v.	pain threshold	18% increase of pain threshold with real acup., effect was partly blocked by naloxone
Lao	*Acupunct. Med.* 1994;**12:** 13–17	RCT patient-blind	10 patients	acup. immediately after surgery vs sham acup.	pain intensity and time until onset of pain	acup. was associated with 57% reduction of pain intensity. Time until onset of pain was 212 min in acup. and 65 min in control group
Scarsella	*Acupunct. Med.* 1994;**12:** 75–77	CCT	200 patients	A) electroacup. at Hegu point B) site-specific points in addition	VAS for pain	in B significantly less postoperative pain than A
Lao	*Oral Surg. Oral Med. Oral Pathol. Oral Radiol. Endod.* 1995;**79:**423–428	RCT patient-blind	19 patients	A) postoperative needle acup. B postoperative shamacup.	time until moderate pain, pain intensity	in A less pain and longer pain-free period

CCT = controlled clinical trial; RCT = randomized clinical trial.

Table 5.3 Controlled clinical trials of acupuncture for back pain

First author	*Reference*	*Design*	*No.*	*Interventions*	*Endpoint*	*Main result*
Edelist	*Can. Anaesth. Soc. J.* 1976; **23:**303–306	RCT patient- and evaluator-blind	30	formula EA vs sham acup.	evaluator's rating of improvement	no intergroup differences
Yue	*Acupunct. Electrother. Res.* 1978;**3:**323–324	RCT evaluator-blind 3 parallel arms	23	formula acup. vs sham acup. vs physiotherapy	pain, range of movement	acup. was superior to physiotherapy but not to sham
Lopacz	*Neurol. Neurochir. Pol.* 1979;**13:**405–409	RCT non-blind 2 parallel arms	34	formula acup. + NaCl injection vs sham electrical stimulation	global assess-ment by physician	acup. superior to controls (NS)
Coan	*Am. J. Chin. Med.* 1980; **8:**181–189	RCT non-blind 2 parallel arms	48	individualized traditional acup. vs waiting-list controls	pain score	pain reduction: acup. 51%, controls 2%
Gunn	*Spine* 1980;**5:**279–291	RCT non-blind 2 parallel arms	46	needling at muscle motor point (mean 7.9) + standard physiotherapy vs physiotherapy alone	pain and work status	needling superior to controls ($P<0.01$)
Gallacchi	*Schweiz. med. Wschr.* 1981; **111:**1360–1366	RCT non-blind 8 parallel arms	~30	formula acup. vs 2 forms of sham acup. vs 5 forms of laser acup.	VAS for pain	all groups improved, no intergroup differences
Duplan	*Sem. Hop. Paris* 1983;**59:** 3109–3114	RCT patient- and evaluator-blind 2 parallel arms	30	formula acup. vs sham acup.	pain VAS on standing 10 minutes, and on resting	acup. superior to sham for severe pain
Macdonald	*Ann. R. Coll. Surg. Engl.* 1983; **65:**44–46	RCT patient- and evaluator-blind 2 parallel arms	16	superficial needling (±EA) vs sham TENS	VAS for pain, etc	pain reduction greater after needling ($P<0.01$)

Table 5.3 continued overleaf

Table 5.3 *continued*

First author	*Reference*	*Design*	*No.*	*Interventions*	*Endpoint*	*Main result*
Mendelson	*Am. J. Med.* 1983;**74:**49–55	RCT patient- and evaluator-blind crossover	77	formula acup. vs lidocaine injections	VAS for pain	no significant difference between groups
Lehmann	*Pain* 1986;**26:**277–290	RCT non-blind 3 parallel arms	53	individualized EA vs TENS vs sham TENS; + education and exercise programme	VAS for pain and disability + physician's assessment	EA superior to TENS (NS); no difference between TENS and sham TENS
Garvey	*Spine* 1989;**14:**962–964	RCT patient- and evaluator-blind 4 parallel arms	63	trigger point needling vs vapocoolant spray + acupressure vs lidocaine injection vs lidocaine + steroid injection	evaluator's rating of improvement	needling and acupressure yielded the best results (NS)
Thomas	*Acta Anaesthesiol. Scand.* 1994;**38:**63–69	RCT non-blind, voluntary crossover, with untreated controls	40	flexible formula acup. vs low frequency EA vs high frequency EA by patient choice (average 6.8) vs waiting-list controls	activity related to pain, mobility, verbal descriptors of pain, patient's assessment of condition	after 6 weeks all EA groups superior to untreated controls (P<0.05); after 6 months this was only the case for low frequency EA

acup = acupuncture; EA = electroacupuncture; NS = not significant; VAS = visual analogue scale.

Of the five sham-controlled studies, one was positive and four were negative. On the basis of these findings, we concluded that data are insufficient to state with certainty that acupuncture is more effective than sham acupuncture or other control interventions in the treatment of neck pain.

Osteoarthritis

Literature searches identified 11 controlled clinical trials of acupuncture for osteoarthritis (Ernst, 1997a). Their key data are summarized in Table 5.5.

The results are highly contradictory. Most trials suffer from significant methodological flaws. The methodologically best studies show no superiority of sham acupuncture over real acupuncture. It was therefore concluded that sham **and** true acupuncture are both equally effective in alleviating symptoms of osteoarthritis, for example through non-specific effects, or they are both equally ineffective. To decide which hypothesis is correct, further research is warranted.

Stroke

Several trials have tested the possibility that acupuncture might be a valuable adjunct for stroke rehabilitation. A systematic review was aimed at determining how solid the collective evidence is (Ernst and White, 1996). Six controlled trials were identified (Table 5.6).

All studies suggested positive effects of acupuncture on functional recovery during the rehabilitation phase following an acute stroke. No trial was free of major methodological flaws. In particular, none had attempted to take possible placebo effects into account. Most trials used electroacupuncture. Electrotherapy is a standard treatment modality in stroke rehabilitation. It is therefore not possible, from these trials, to determine pure acupuncture effects. Conceivably, the promising clinical results were a result of the electrotherapeutic element or non-specific effects. It was concluded that the evidence is encouraging yet, at present, far from convincing. Future studies are warranted; in particular they should attempt to define to what extent the apparent effectiveness is due to non-specific (placebo) effects or due to specific effects of acupuncture.

Smoking cessation

Because acupuncture is often advocated as an aid for smoking cessation, this systematic review and meta-analysis was aimed at determining whether or not it is effective for this indication (White *et al.*, 1999). Ten sham-controlled, patient-blind RCTs were located (Table 5.7). The methodological quality of these studies was satisfactory on average.

Table 5.4 Controlled trials of acupuncture for neck pain

First author	*Reference*	*Design*	*No.*	*Interventions (sessions)*	*Endpoint*	*Main result*
Gallacchi	*Schweiz. Med. Wschr.* 1981;**111**(37):1360–1366	RCT parallel groups	45	formula acup A) sham acup B) non-point needling	pain (VAS) no follow-up	a) acup. = sham b) acup. = non-point
Coan	*Am. J. Chin. Med.* 1982;**9:**326–332	RCT parallel groups	30	classical individual acup waiting list	pain (hour/day) follow-up 3 months	acup. significant > nil
Junnila	*Am. J. Acupunct.* 1982;**10:**259–262	RCT parallel groups	44	formula acup sham: pricked with finger-nail	pain (VAS) follow-up 1 month	acup. significant > sham
Loy	*Med. J. Aust.* 1983;**2:**32–34	RCT parallel groups	60	points from list physiotherapy (short-wave, traction)	ROM, pain relief percent follow-up 6 weeks	acup. 87% relief physiotherapy 54% relief no stats
Petrie	*Clin. Exp. Rheumatol.* 1983;**1:** 333–335	RCT parallel groups	13	formula acup sham TENS	pain relief scale no follow-up	acup. significant > sham TENS
Emery	*Br. J. Rheumatol.* 1986;**25:** 132–133	RCT crossover	20	formula + EA sham: needle-prick only	pain (VAS) no follow-up	acup. = sham
Kreczi	*Acupunct. Electrother. Res.* 1986;**11:**207–216	RCT crossover (short-term)	42	laser acup sham laser	pain (VAS) follow-up 24 hours	laser significant > mock laser up to 6 hours laser = mock laser at 24 hours
Petrie	*Br. J. Rheumatol.* 1986;**25:** 271–275	RCT parallel groups	25	formula acup sham TENS	pain (VAS) follow-up 1 week	acup. = sham
Ceccherelli	*Clin. J. Pain* 1989;**5:**301–304	RCT parallel groups	27	laser to tender + acup. points sham laser	pain (McGill) follow-up 3 months	laser significant >placebo

Lundeberg	*Pain Clinic* 1991;**4:**155–161	RCT parallel groups (short-term)	58	A) formula, manual acup B) EA 2 Hz C) EA 80 Hz D) superficial needling	pain (VAS) follow-up 140 mins	acup. = sham = EA 2 Hz = EA 80 Hz
Thomas	*Am. J. Chin. Med.* 1991;**19:** 95–100	RCT crossover (short-term)	176	formula acup A) superficial acup B) diazepam C) placebo diazepam	sensory & affective pain (VAS) follow-up 2 hours	a) acup = superficial acup. b) acup = diazepam c) acup sig > placebo diazepam
Kisiel	*Sjukgymnasten* 1996;**12:** S24–S31	RCT parallel groups	19	flexible formula acup physiotherapy	pain (VAS) follow-up 6 months	acup. = physiotherapy
David	Unpublished	RCT parallel groups	70	formula + tender points physiotherapy	pain (VAS) follow-up 6 months	acup. = physiotherapy
Irnich	Unpublished	RCT crossover	68	local and distant points from list A) dry needling B) sham laser	ROM, pain	a) acup. slightly > dry needling b) acup significant > sham laser

acup = acupuncture; EA = electroacupuncture; OA = osteoarthritis; ROM = range of movement; stats = statistics; VAS = visual analogue scale.

Table 5.5 Controlled trials of acupuncture for osteoarthritis

First author	*Reference*	*Design*	*No.*	*Interventions*	*Endpoint*	*Main result*
Gaw	*N. Engl. J. Med.* 1975; **293:**375–378	RCT double-blind, sham-controlled	40 patients/ various sites	formula acup. vs acup. at placebo points, once/week,	tenderness, subjective report	both groups improved, no intergroup differences
Coan	*Am. J. Chin. Med.* 1982;**9:**326–332	RCT	30 patients/ cervical	electroacup. and moxibustion to traditional points (2–3/week for 12 weeks) vs no treatment controls	pain	acup. group 40% pain reduction, controls 2% pain increase
Junnila	*Am. J. Acupunct.* 1982;**10:**341–347	crossover trial, non-random, not blinded	32 patients/ large joints	formula acup., individualized frequency of treatment vs piroxicam (20 mg/day), for 4 months	pain by VAS	at end of treatment period significantly less pain in acup. group. 2 months later effect sustained
Loy	*Med. J. Aust.* 1983; **2:**32–34	controlled clinical trial	60 patients cervical	formula electroacup. vs physiotherapy for 4 weeks	subjective improvement and ROM	acup. group showed numerically better results
Petrie	*Clin. Exp. Rheumatol.* 1983;**1:**333–335	RCT	13 patients cervical	formula acup. vs sham TENS, twice weekly for 4 weeks	pain	significantly greater pain relief in acup. group
Petrie	*Br. J. Rheumatol.* 1986;**25:**271–275	RCT single-blind	25 patients cervical	formula acup. vs TENS for 4 weeks	pain, function, analgesics use	at end of treatment period and at 1 month follow-up no intergroup differences
Ammer	*Wien. Med. Wochenschr.* 1988;**22:** 566–569	controlled clinical trial	14 patients/ knee	formula acup. vs physiotherapy for 4 weeks	pain and other symptoms	some improvement in both groups but significantly more with physiotherapy
Petrou	*Scand. J. Acupunct.* 1988;**3:**112–115	RCT, sham-controlled	31 patients/ knee	formula vs sham acup. 3 times/week for 3 weeks	pain by VAS	significantly more improvement in real compared to sham acup.

Dickens	*Compl. Med. Res.* 1989;**3:**5–8	RCT single-blind	12 patients/ trapezio-metacarpal joint	formula acup. vs sham TENS 3 times/week for 2 weeks	pain	acup. was numerically superior
Thomas	*Am. J. Chin. Med.* 1991;**14:**95–100	randomized crossover trial	44 patients/ cervical	formula vs sham acup., each session = 40 min, no. of sessions not mentioned	pain by VAS	both groups improved; no intergroup differences
Christensen	*Acta Anaesthesiol. Scand.* 1992;**36:** 519–525	RCT, single-blind	29 patients/ knee(s)	formula acup. 2 times/week for 3 weeks vs no treatment group	analgesic use, pain function (ROM)	all variable were significantly more improved in acup. group
Takeda	*Arthritis Care Res.* 1994;**7:**118–122	RCT, double-blind, sham-controlled	40 patients/ knee(s)	formula vs sham acup. 3 times/week for 3 weeks	2 validated pain rating scales, pain threshold at knee	both groups improved, no intergroup differences
Fink	*Forsch. Kompl. Med.* 1996:(abstract)	RCT, single-blind, sham-controlled	67 patients/ hip	formula vs sham acup.	pain by VAS, ROM	both groups improved, no intergroup differences

RCT = randomized controlled trial; ROM = range of motion; TENS = transcutaneous nerve stimulation; VAS = visual analogue scale.

Table 5.6 Controlled clinical trials of acupuncture for stroke

First author	*Reference*	*Design*	*No.*	*Interventions*[1]	*Endpoint*	*Main result*
Zou	*Chin. J. Mod. Dev. Trad. Med.* 1990;**10:**195–202	RCT, open	63 patients with cerebral infarction	'calan' (5 mg) 4 tablets/day	functional recovery	'the therapeutic effect in the acup. group was better'
Hu	*Neuroepidemiology* 1993;**12:**106–113	RCT, open	30 acute stroke patients	standard medical and rehabilitative treatment	Barthel index	experimental group had significantly less deficit on days 28 and 90
Johansson	*Neurology* 1993;**43:** 2189–2192	RCT, open	78 subacute stroke patients	standard medical and rehabilitative treatments	Barthel index, activities of daily living	experimental group had significantly better outcome at 1 and 3 months. Also better quality of life
Li	*Chen Tzu Yen Chiu Acu. Res.* 1994;**19:**4–7	RCT, open	108 patients with stroke	standard medical care	functional recovery	experimental group fared significantly better than controls
Liang	*J. Trad. Chin. Med.* 1994; **14:**110–114	controlled trial, open	101 patients with stroke	information incomplete	functional recovery	'the therapeutic effects were encouraging'
Sallström	*Tidskrift. Den. Norske Laegefor.* 1995;**115:** 2884–2887	RCT, open	45 subacute stroke patients	standard medical and rehabilitative treatments	motor function, activities of daily living	experimental group had better outcome and quality of life after 6 weeks

RCT = randomized controlled trial.
[1]Experimental groups received regular acupuncture in addition.

The combined odds ratio for smoking cessation directly at the end of a series of acupuncture was 1.2 (CI 0.98–1.48). After 6 months it was 1.2 (CI 0.82–2.01) and after 12 months it was 1.3 (CI 0.73–1.46). No particular aspect could be identified that rendered one form of acupuncture more successful than another. On the basis of this evidence, it was concluded that acupuncture is no more effective than sham acupuncture for smoking cessation.

Weight loss

Finally, a systematic review was performed of all randomized, sham-controlled clinical trials of acupuncture for weight reduction (Ernst, 1997b). Four studies met the inclusion/exclusion criteria (Table 5.1) and were included for analysis. All studies were burdened with serious methodological flaws.

The results of the four trials were highly contradictory (Table 5.8). Two relatively rigorous studies demonstrated no effect, while the two less rigorous studies suggested some benefit. Thus, no clear picture emerged as to the efficacy of acupuncture for this indication. It was concluded that claims that acupuncture is effective for weight loss are not based on the evidence from well-performed clinical trials.

Discussion

This overview of our own systematic reviews and meta-analyses indicates that reasonably good evidence exists for acupuncture to be effective in alleviating dental pain (Ernst and Pittler, 1998) and low back pain (Ernst and White, 1998). For stroke, the evidence is uniformly positive but unconvincing because of methodological problems (Ernst and White, 1996). The trial data are contradictory for neck pain (White and Ernst, 1999). For osteoarthritis, the evidence is negative but, because of methodological problems, not convincingly so (Ernst, 1997a). For smoking cessation the data are convincingly negative (White *et al.*, 1999).

Other research groups have performed similar analyses and contributed important information in this area. Ter Riet and colleagues (1990) concluded that, for various forms of addiction, acupuncture is not more effective than sham acupuncture. Vickers (1996) found in his systematic review that acupuncture/acupressure is convincingly more effective than sham interventions to alleviate the symptoms of nausea and vomiting due to various aetiologies. Linde and colleagues (1997) conducted a 'Cochrane Review' of acupuncture for asthma and found some encouraging evidence but, overall, had to draw a cautious conclusion. A review of all Medline-listed clinical trials of acupuncture for inflammatory rheumatic diseases (predominantly rheumatoid arthritis) found not a single study that would meet today's accepted methodological standards (Lautenschlager, 1997). The author therefore concludes that 'acupuncture cannot be recommended for treatment of these diseases'.

Table 5.7 Controlled clinical trials of acupuncture for smoking cessation

First author	*Reference*	*Design*[1]	*No.*	*Interventions*	*Endpoint*	*Main result*
Clavel	*Rev. Epidém. Santé Publ.* 1992;**40:** 187–190	sham-controlled, single-blind RCT 4 parallel groups	996	A) facial points B) sham points both with nicotine or placebo gum	cessation at 13 months	no significant difference between groups
Gilbey	*Am. J. Acupunct.* 1977; **5:**239–247	sham-controlled, single-blind RCT	92	A) auricular points B) sham points	cessation at 3 months	no significant difference between groups
Gillams	*Practitioner* 1984;**228:** 341–344	sham-controlled, single-blind RCT 3 parallel groups	81	A) auricular points B) sham points C) behaviour therapy	cessation at 6 months	no significant difference between groups
Lacroix	*Ann. Méd. Interne* 1977; **128:**405–408	sham-controlled, single-blind RCT	117	A) facial points B) sham points	cessation at 2 weeks	acup. significantly more effective than sham ($P < 0.01$)
Lagrue	*Nouv. Presse Méd.* 1977;**9:**966	sham-controlled, single-blind RCT	154	A) facial points B) sham points	cessation at 1 week	no significant difference between groups
Lamontagne	*Can. Med. Assoc. J.* 1980;**5:**787–790	sham-controlled, single-blind RCT 3 parallel groups	75	A) auricular acup. B) body acup. C) waiting list control	cessation at 6 months	no significant difference between groups
Martin	*N. Z. Med. J.* 1981;**93:** 421–423	sham-controlled, single-blind RCT 4 parallel groups	260	A) auricular points B) as 1 + EA C) sham points D) as 3 + EA	cessation at 6 months	no significant difference between groups
Parker	*Am. J. Acupunct.* 1977; **5:**363–366	sham-controlled, single-blind RCT	41	A) auricular points B) as 1 + EA C) sham points D) as 3 + EA	cessation at 6 weeks	no significant difference between groups

Steiner	*Am. J. Chin. Med.* 1982; **10:**107–121	sham-controlled, single-blind RCT	22	A) body + auricular points B) sham points	cessation at 4 weeks	no significant difference between groups
Vandevenne	*Sem. Hôp. Paris* 1985; **61:**2155–2160	sham-controlled, single-blind RCT	200	A) body + facial points B) sham points	cessation at 12 months	no significant difference between groups

[1]Two parallel groups unless stated otherwise.
EA = electroacupuncture.

Table 5.8 Controlled clinical trials of acupuncture/acupressure for weight loss

First author	*Reference*	*Design*	*No.*	*Interventions*	*Endpoint*	*Main result*
Giller	*Am. J. Acupunct.* 1975;**3:**151–153	RCT with 4 parallel groups	120 volunteers	permanent needles at: 1. lung point 2. stomach point 3. hunger point each for 6 weeks	hunger	groups 1, 2 and 4: 20% experienced body weight reduction and reported hunger abatement group 3: 70% had such results
Mok	*Am. J. Clin. Nutr.* 1976;**29:**832–835	RCT with 3 treatment periods (crossover)	24 obese volunteers	permanent needles at: 1. unilateral ear points 2. bilateral ear points 3. sham points each for 3 weeks	body weight	no intergroup differences in body weight. Subjectively less hunger in verum phases
Allison	*Int. J. Obesity* 1995; **19:**653–658	RCT with 2 parallel groups	96 obese volunteers	1. acupressure at ear point 2. acupressure at wrist (placebo) each for 12 weeks	body weight	small weight loss in both groups, no intergroup difference
Shafshak[1]	*Am. J. Clin. Med.* 1995;**13:**15–25	RCT with 3 parallel groups	30 obese women	acup. at: 1. hunger point 2 stomach point 3. placebo point 5 sessions/week for 3 weeks + hypocaloric diet	hunger	70%, 80% and 20% of groups 1, 2 and 3 respectively, complied with diet. This was accompanied with respective weight loss

RCT = randomized controlled trial.
[1]The author reports two further studies, both of which were not placebo/sham-controlled.

According to a recent UK survey, acupuncturists most frequently attend chronic or acute musculoskeletal problems, other painful conditions, emotional problems as well as people wanting to stop smoking (Dale, 1997). In this survey, there were surprisingly few differences between medical and non-medical acupuncturists. A similar investigation, conducted on traditional Chinese acupuncturists in the UK, found that the conditions treated most often were musculoskeletal problems, emotional/psychological disorders, ENT disorders, low energy, digestive disorders, headache and migraine (Wadlow and Peringer, 1996). A survey of British medical acupuncturists suggested that the most frequent indications were general pain, musculoskeletal pain, gynaecological disorders, dermatological diseases and addictions (Hayhoe and Box, 1997). Thus we can be confident that this overview of meta-analyses and systematic reviews covers many of the conditions regularly seen by acupuncturists in daily practice.

Caution is required when interpreting the above findings. One has to bear in mind that publication bias could have contributed to false positive (or negative) findings (Ernst and Pittler, 1997). One should also remember that absence of evidence should never be equated with evidence of absence of an effect.

The above systematic reviews and meta-analyses had to be based on certain assumptions. For instance, it had to be assumed that one form of acupuncture is essentially the same as another (in most cases, there were simply not enough studies to attempt more subtle differentiations). Almost certainly, this is a gross over-simplification. It is clearly possible that electroacupuncture differs significantly from traditional needle acupuncture and that Chinese (individualized) acupuncture leads to different effects than formula or trigger point acupuncture. As soon as sufficient trial data become available, comparisons by type of acupuncture need to clarify this issue.

In those cases where 'real' acupuncture was compared to sham acupuncture, it was assumed that sham acupuncture is inactive and that one form of sham (e.g. needling non-acupuncture points) is essentially the same as another form of sham acupuncture (e.g. touching the skin of a blinded patient with a cocktail stick). This assumption could well be wrong (Vincent and Lewith, 1995; Ernst and White, 1997). We need more data on this issue, more trials to do meaningful subanalyses of different sham-interventions and possibly a consensus of the acupuncture world as to what exactly constitutes an ideal sham.

It is possible, on the basis of the totality of the above evidence, to categorize indications as to the soundness of supporting evidence (Table 5.9). It is interesting, however, to note that 'conclusively shown to be effective' does not necessarily mean that acupuncture is useful for this condition. Acupuncture may, for instance, alleviate dental pain, but in clinical practice there may be other analgesic treatments that could be simpler, less expensive and more effective. Similarly, the fact that acupuncture is not more effective than sham acupuncture for smoking cessation does not mean that it is entirely useless. In fact, it is associated with a sizeable placebo effect, which leads to immediate cessation in about 35% of all patients. Thus its non-specific effects could well be worth

Table 5.9 The evidence* regarding acupuncture

Conclusively positive	*Inconclusive*	*Conclusively negative*
dental pain low back pain nausea/vomiting	experimental pain neck pain headache/migraine osteoarthritis inflammatory rheumatic diseases stroke addictions asthma	smoking cessation weight loss

*based on systematic reviews/meta-analyses of RCTs

exploiting in clinical practice. One precondition for using acupuncture in this way would be that it is reasonably safe. For a discussion of this topic, the reader is referred to the following chapter.

The largest category in Table 5.9 is formed by conditions for which the evidence is presently inconclusive. It is interesting to note that this can be the case for different reasons. For stroke, the evidence is unanimously positive but the trials are methodologically flawed. For osteoarthritis, there are rigorous trials available, but they are highly contradictory as to their results. Thus 'inconclusive evidence' can mean more than just one thing.

Perhaps the only conclusion that, on the basis of the above data, can be generalized is that we need more rigorous trials if we want to advance our knowledge in this area. Regardless of indication, many of the existing trials are methodologically flawed. We therefore repeat our suggestion (Ernst and White, 1997) that good acupuncture research must be the result of a team of experts working together. A minimum requirement would be expertise in the practice of acupuncture, in the condition to be treated, in statistics and in trial methodology. It is obvious that clinical acupuncture research is more complex than, for instance, the investigation of drug treatments. To meet this complexity adequate funds would be a 'conditio sine qua non'. Unfortunately, many of the normal sources for medical research have, in the past, been less than generous for acupuncture research. If we want to establish the true value of acupuncture the unfortunate funding situation would need to change dramatically.

References

Dale, J. (1997). Acupuncture practice in the UK. Part 1: report of a survey. *Comp. Ther. Med.*, **5,** 215–220.

Ernst, E. (1997a) Acupuncture as a symptomatic treatment of osteoarthritis. A systematic review. *Scand. J. Rheumatol.*, **26,** 444–447.

Ernst, E. (1997b) Acupuncture for weight reduction? A systematic review. *Wien. Klin. Wochenschr.*, **109,** 60–62.

Ernst, E. and Pittler, M. H. (1997) Alternative therapy bias. *Nature*, **385,** 480.

Ernst, E. and Pittler, M. H. (1998) The effectiveness of acupuncture in treating acute dental pain: a systematic review. *Br. Dent. J.*, **184,** 443–447.

Ernst, E. and White, A. R. (1996) Acupuncture as an adjuvant therapy in stroke rehabilitation. *Wien. Med. Wochenschr.*, **146,** 556–558.

Ernst, E. and White, A. R. (1997) A review of problems in clinical acupuncture research. *Am. J. Chin. Med.*, **25,** 3–11.

Ernst, E. and White, A. R. (1998) Acupuncture for back pain: a meta-analysis of randomized controlled trials. *Arch. Int. Med. 1998,* **158**, 2235–2241.

Hayhoe, S. and Box, H. (1997) A questionnaire on medical acupuncture practice. *Acupunct. Med.*, **15,** 96–99.

Jadad, A. R., Moore, R. A., Carrol, D. *et al.* (1996) Assessing the quality of reports of randomized clinical trials: is blinding necessary? *Contr. Clin. Trials*, **17,** 1–12.

Lautenschläger, J. (1997). Akupunktur bei der Behandlung entzündlich – rheumatischer Erkrankungen. *Z. Rheumatol.*, **56,** 8–20.

Linde, K., Jobst, K. and Panton, J. (1997). Acupuncture for the treatment of asthma bronchiale. *Cochrane Library*, (2), 1.

NIH (1997).Consensus Development Statement: Acupuncture. 3–5 November.

Ter Riet, G., Kleijnen, J. and Knipschild, P. (1990) A meta-analysis of studies into the effect of acupuncture on addiction. *Br. J. Gen. Pract.*, **40**, 379–382.

Vickers, A. J. (1996) Can acupuncture have specific effects on health? A systematic review of acupuncture anti-emesis trials. *J. R. Soc. Med.*, **89,** 303–311.

Vincent, C. and Lewith, G. (1995) Placebo controls for acupuncture studies. *J. R. Soc. Med.*, **88,** 199–202.

Wadlow, G. and Peringer E. (1996) Retrospective survey of patients and practitioners of traditional Chinese acupuncture in the UK. *Comp. Ther. Med.*, **4**, 1–7.

White, A. R. and Ernst, E. (1998) Assessing the adequacy of acupuncture treatments: a trial of a new method. *Alt. Ther. Health Med.*, **4**, 66–71.

White, A. R. and Ernst, E. (1999). A systematic review of randomized controlled trials of acupuncture for neck pain. *Rheumatology*, **38**, 143–147.

White, A. R., Resch, K. L. and Ernst, E. (1999) A meta-analysis of acupuncture techniques for smoking cessation. *Tobacco Control* (in press).

6

Adverse effects of acupuncture

Hagen Rampes and Elmar Peuker

Introduction

In common with many of the complementary therapies, acupuncture is perceived as being natural and holistic. Because of these perceptions, there is a myth that acupuncture is completely safe. Since 1965, publications have repeatedly reported life-threatening incidents in association with acupuncture treatment. These reports do not usually appear in the journals for acupuncturists, but in those of the specialists who manage the complications.

Recent literature surveys (Rampes and James, 1995; Ernst and White, 1997b; Peuker and Filler, 1997a) have identified all reports of adverse reactions of acupuncture. The databases searched included: the Complementary & Alternative Therapies database, Premedline and Medline [1966–1998], Psyndex [1977–1998], Psychlit [1974–1998], UMI Dissertation Abstracts [1981–1997], Ciscom [1995–1998], Healthstar [1977–1998] and Current Contents [1995–1998]. Further articles were identified by extensive cross referencing. Articles were included if adverse effects, complications and potentially life-threatening incidents in association with acupuncture treatment were reported, and excluded if investigations were not performed on human subjects. All English, German or French language articles identified were studied in detail. In conclusion, over 300 instances of serious complications were reported world-wide over a 30-year period.

Adverse effects

In general, the reported adverse effects of acupuncture therapy can be categorized in the following groups:

- Delayed or missed diagnosis.
- Deterioration of disorder under treatment.
- Pain.
- Vegetative reactions.
- Bacterial and viral infection.
- Trauma of tissues and organs.
- Miscellaneous.

Delayed or missed diagnosis (i.e. orthodox diagnostic categories)

This first topic deals with a more general problem: the diagnostic skills of the acupuncturists. A significant number of acupuncturists are not medically qualified. There can be no doubt that several diseases are curable in their early stages but may end fatally if diagnosis is delayed or missed. A patient was reported as dying of a myocardial infarction 5–6 hours after acupuncture for pains in the back and the left arm (Bostrom and Rossner, 1990). One of the problems in most of the case reports referred to is the attribution of causality. It may well have been that this patient had referred pain from myocardial infarction and the practitioner missed the diagnosis and inappropriately treated the patient with acupuncture.

The disregard of orthodox diagnostic categories might represent an indirect risk of acupuncture (Ernst, 1995). Twenty-five per cent of American patients, who sought care from a physician for a serious health problem, also had used an unconventional therapy for the same problem. Many of them (70%) did not report using an unconventional therapy to their doctors (Eisenberg *et al.*, 1993).

Deterioration of disorder under treatment

There has been one reported case (Carron *et al.*, 1974) of an asthmatic who discontinued all his medication while undergoing acupuncture for his illness. He progressively deteriorated and developed status asthmaticus. This is not an adverse effect of acupuncture, of course, but a consequence of inadvisedly discontinuing medication.

Pain

Patients often expect pain during acupuncture. Traditionally a strong needling sensation (DeQi) is obtained (Buck, 1986). This is a characteristic sensation that arises when an acupuncture point is successfully stimulated. It is distinct from the simple pin-prick sensation and is variously described as dull, numb, swelling, sore or radiating along a limb to nearby acupuncture points. It may be experienced as pain by some patients, especially if they have not been forewarned or if their pain threshold is low. Persistent pain following acupuncture has been reported (Lapeer and Monga, 1988). A 42-year-old female received electroacupuncture for an acute attack of migraine. Needles were inserted bilaterally at large intestine (LI) 4 and a current of 60 mA at a frequency of 6 Hz (continuous waveform) was applied for 20 minutes. She developed tingling in both hands and her right arm following the treatment. This progressed to a severe pain in her forearm and paraesthesia in her right thumb. This pain lasted for several days and resolved following a course of diflunisal 500 mg for 10 days. The authors concluded that the pain may have been due to either an irritation of the superficial branch of the radial nerve and/or the digital branch of the median nerve. The authors discussed other possibilities such as carpal tunnel syndrome or radiculopathy, but unfortunately the patient refused to have nerve conduction studies. Another case report (Brougham, 1988) concerned a 45-year-old man who had back pain and was found to have normal investigations. He received acupuncture treatment at a tender site in the lower thoracic spine and at distal points. He returned a few days later with a marked worsening of his back pain. Repeat investigations revealed a chest X-ray which had a suspicious lesion in the ninth thoracic vertebra. The patient died 5 weeks later from multiple secondaries.

Vegetative reactions

Syncope

A prospective cohort study of patients receiving acupuncture at the Centre for Traditional Medicine of Veterans General Hospital, Taipei in Taiwan reported that 0.19% (55 out of 28 285 acupuncture procedures) resulted in syncope (Chen *et al.*, 1990). Of those that had syncope, 35 were male and 17 female. Mean age was 45.2 (± 16.7) with bimodal distribution of the young (20–29) and the elderly (60–69). Patients who experienced syncope or 'needle fainting' were all in a seated or upright posture when they received acupuncture. Occurrences of syncope were within 2–10 minutes of needle insertion. None of the patients developed complete loss of consciousness and all recovered without sequelae. The vaso-vagal fainting episodes usually occurred in young male and elderly patients in the early phase of the treatment. There have been case reports (Rajanna, 1983; Verma and Khamesra, 1989) of syncope following acupuncture. Two patients (Hayhoe and Pitt, 1987) proceeded to have convulsions, which were probably hypoxia induced.

Drowsiness

Drowsiness is common during and after acupuncture; in fact acupuncture can be soporific. There is thus a potential risk where patients driving home after treatment may be a danger to themselves and others. A study (Brattberg, 1986) was conducted of 122 consecutive patients who received acupuncture at a pain clinic in Sandviken Hospital, Norway. Needles were inserted at the site of pain and manipulated (4–20 needles). Fifty six per cent were deemed to be a significant traffic hazard had they driven a car home directly after the treatment. Excessive drowsiness with the risk of falling asleep was experienced by 36% of patients. Ten per cent fell asleep after getting home. Twenty five per cent were moderately drowsy even after their third acupuncture treatment. Twenty three per cent were unaffected by the first three treatments and only became drowsy in subsequent treatments. The study made no mention of patients' concurrent medication and whether such medication may have contributed to or enhanced acupuncture-induced drowsiness. The authors were unable to predict which patient would become drowsy or when in the course of the treatment this drowsiness may appear. They recommended that a warning against driving a car while undergoing acupuncture treatment should therefore be issued to all patients. It is worthwhile noting that doctors are obliged to inform patients about medication that may impair their ability to drive or operate machinery.

Bacterial and viral infection

Septicaemia

There have been reports of septicaemia (Doutsu *et al.*, 1986) resulting from *Staphylococcus aureus*. Two patients, who had complex past medical histories and were debilitated, died following acupuncture treatment with press needles (Pierik, 1982). These are small needles for indwelling use in auricular therapy and may be left in place for 1 week or longer to produce continued effect. In one case (Izatt and Fairman, 1977) acupuncture around a knee joint resulted in septicaemia with fulminant disseminated intravascular coagulation. Harada *et al.* (1997) reported the case of an 80-year-old male who developed a toxic shock-like syndrome and superficial fasciitis, multiple organ failure with shock after acupuncture treatment of both legs. Group A streptococcus was detected from culture. The patient recovered from the disease after amputation of the involved leg and antibiotic therapy.

Endocarditis

Bacterial endocarditis (Jefferys *et al.*, 1983; Lee and Mcilwain, 1985; Scheel *et al.*, 1992) has been reported in three cases. Patients who had prosthetic heart valves underwent acupuncture involving the use of press needles for a number of days. The reports of endocarditis raise important questions about patients' suitability for acupuncture. In the correspondence following the first report of endocarditis (Jefferys *et al.*, 1983), Cheng (1983) criticized prophylactic measures suggested by the authors of the report. It had been suggested that antibiotic prophylaxis be used in all patients with cardiac lesions undergoing acupuncture. However, acupuncture is not a single procedure, but entails a course of treatment; therefore it would be impracticable and uneconomical to use antibiotics for each acupuncture session. The reported cases of endocarditis occurred with the use of press needles, retained in the skin for up to a week. It would be strongly advised for patients who have prosthetic or damaged heart valves not to have acupuncture involving press needles.

Perichondritis

Auricular acupuncture lends itself to the use of press needles. The commonest use of press needles is for the treatment of smoking and obesity. These needles are inserted at known auricular acupuncture points or at any tender areas of the ear. Press needles were implicated in all the reports of perichondritis except one case where intradermal needles were inappropriately used (Allison and Kravitz, 1975; Baltimore and Moloy, 1976; Trautermann and Trautermann, 1981; Davis and Powell, 1985; Savage-Jones, 1985; Warwick-Brown and Richards, 1986; Gilbert, 1987; Johansen and Nielsen, 1990; Sorensen, 1990). Perichondritis is a serious adverse reaction. The treatment may entail parenteral antibiotics and surgical intervention. Some of the patients were left with a cosmetically deformed ear following treatment. A recent litigation case (Evans, 1989) involved a young female who received ear acupuncture for rheumatoid arthritis. The ear lobe was cleaned with a swab before the needle was inserted. The needle was left in situ for 6 days. The needle site became infected. She was prescribed fucidin and the ear was dressed. The infection progressed and developed into a perichondritis requiring three surgical operations. The patient was left with an unsightly cauliflower ear. Unfortunately none of the case reports of perichondritis had sufficient detail to scrutinize the method of acupuncture. For example, what aseptic technique (the adequate disinfection of the skin and avoidance of handling the sterile needles), if any, was practised? Were patients instructed to stimulate the retained press needles? How long were the needles retained in the ear? As the wound created by needle insertion needs about 5–7 days to heal, the use of press needles may not be necessary at all.

Hepatitis

Doctors visiting China who have seen the practice of acupuncture in a rural setting have expressed concern (Alexander *et al.*, 1974) at the lack of aseptic technique. Some have speculated (Li and Shiang, 1980; Conn, 1988) about a link between the use of acupuncture and the high prevalence of hepatitis and hepatocellular carcinoma in China.

There have been definitive reports (Hussain, 1974; Negro *et al.*, 1977; Kobler *et al.*, 1979; De Galocsy *et al.*, 1982; Schmid *et al.*, 1984; Dominguez *et al.*, 1985; Garcia-Bengoechea *et al.*, 1985; Moro-Aguado *et al.*, 1985; Batisse, 1986; Stryker *et al.*, 1986; Kiyosawa *et al.*, 1987; Alexis *et al.*, 1988; Kent *et al.*, 1988; Slater *et al.*, 1988) of dissemination of hepatitis B. There was a recent report of three cases of hepatitis B between December 1990 and October 1992 from an acupuncture clinic in south west London. (Communicable Disease Surveillance Centre of the PHLS, 1992). The first report in the UK (Communicable Diseases Surveillance Centre of the PHLS, 1977; Boxall, 1978) was influential because practitioners switched over to using sterile disposable needles and public health supervision improved. A practitioner was noted to have appallingly poor hygienic technique. He was seen to handle the needle points before and after insertion. He infected 36 patients and himself became infected through a needlestick injury. His technique was also unusual in that he used hollow needles. Other well-documented hepatitis outbreaks occurred where standard solid acupuncture needles were used and the infections were all attributed to failure to adhere to strict aseptic technique. One practitioner dipped his used acupuncture needles into calendula ointment (Hussain,

1974), another used a disinfectant (Stryker *et al.*, 1986) to clean his needles; neither technique is effective to sterilize the needles.

The transmission of hepatitis B and other blood-borne infections via acupuncture needles can be prevented by using sterile disposable needles. The need to autoclave reusable needles and the fact that these needles become blunt with repeated use are the main disadvantages of using such needles. It is far more convenient and relatively inexpensive to use sterile disposable stainless steel acupuncture needles. We recommend that the use of sterile disposable needles should be mandatory.

The British Blood Transfusion Service screening of potential blood donors inquires about acupuncture. If acupuncture has been performed by a registered medical practitioner or physiotherapist, or an acupuncturist registered with the British Acupuncture Council, the donor is accepted. If acupuncture was administered by others then the donor is asked to wait 6 months (HMSO, 1989). The German Red Cross inquires about acupuncture therapy too. If acupuncture was performed with sterile disposable needles by a doctor, the donor is accepted, otherwise he or she has to wait for 6 months.

AIDS

There has been much publicity about the acquired immune deficiency syndrome and speculation whether acupuncture can transmit the human immunodeficiency virus (HIV). There have been no proven cases, although we have identified one reported case (Vittecoq *et al.*, 1989b) suggesting that acupuncture was implicated. This was a 17-year-old French male who did not have any risk factors for HIV infection. He received acupuncture for tendinitis and subsequently developed the symptoms of AIDS. The ensuing correspondence concluded that the case report was speculative and there was insufficient information to attribute causality (Chamberland *et al.*, 1989; Vittecoq *et al.*, 1989b). In a study (Castro *et al.*, 1988) by the Centre for Diseases Control, USA, cases of AIDS in patients who did not have any apparent risk factors were thoroughly investigated; two of 2059 were found to have had acupuncture before the symptoms developed.

The UK government produced AIDS information leaflets suggesting that acupuncture needles may transmit HIV (HMSO, 1986). However, there is no definite evidence that acupuncture needles have caused HIV transmission. The risk to the practitioner from needlestick injury when treating a patient who is carrying HIV may be more important.

Other infections

There have been isolated reports of spinal infection (Hadden and Swanson, 1982) and a case of suspected osteomyelitis (Jones and Cross, 1980). A 48-year-old female expressed signs of meningeal irritation after having received several lumbar acupunctures within 1 week for back pain. Bacterial meningitis was diagnosed from cerebrospinal fluid examinations (Chen *et al.*, 1997). Recently a glenohumeral pyarthrosis following acupuncture treatment was reported (Kirschenbaum and Rizzo, 1997). Arthrocentesis produced thick purulent fluid and *Staph. aureus* was isolated in the cultures.

Trauma of tissues and organs

Cardiac tamponade

Six cases of injuries to the heart and the pericardium have been described so far in the scientific literature (Schiff, 1965; Nieda *et al.*, 1973; Cheng, 1991; Hasegawa *et al.*, 1991; Halvorsen *et al.*, 1995; Kataoka, 1997), two of which ended fatally (Schiff, 1965; Halvorsen *et al.*, 1995). One was a result of self acupuncture (Schiff, 1965). The needle had penetrated the pericardium and caused cardiac tamponade. In an acupuncturist-induced fatality in Norway (Halvorsen *et al.*, 1995), a 40-year-old woman died after treatment for fibromyalgia using conception vessel (CV) 17, a mid-sternal point. The patient complained of chest pain and died about 2 hours after the insertion of the needle. Post-mortem revealed the cause of death to be cardiac tamponade, following a puncture wound in the right ventricle. The responsibility for such injuries lies, among other things, in ignorance of the foramen sternale. This common congenital abnormality exists in approximately 5–8% of the population. It is usually located in the level of the fourth intercostal space, i.e. precisely at the acupuncture point CV 17 (Figure 6.1).

It cannot be identified by standard chest X-ray. Using CT scanning, Stark (1985) found this variation in 4.8% of his sample. Cooper *et al.*

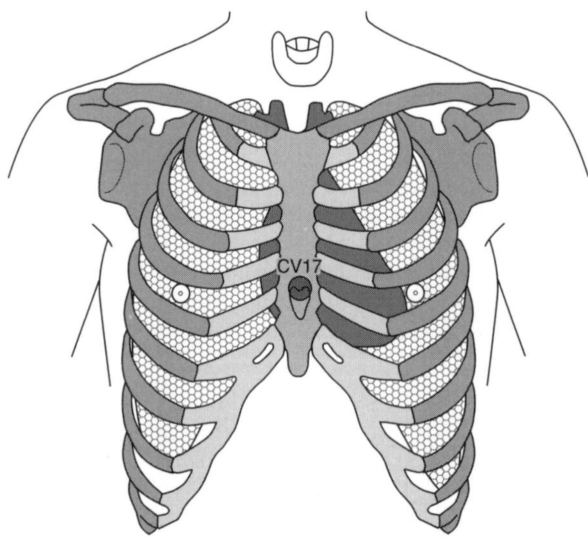

Figure 6.1 Scheme of the chest with foramen sternale underlying CV 17: acupuncture point conception vessel 17.

(1988) detected a foramen sternale in 6.7% of all autopsies he performed. Schratter *et al.* (1997) evaluated 100 chest CT scans with reference to the incidence of the foramen sternale and its features. They distinguished four types of this anomaly, varying from incomplete retraction of the sternal cortex to complete foraminal defects. A foramen sternale was present in 8%, and of sufficient size in 6% to constitute a risk of complications during medical interventions. The distance between the surface of the skin and the posterior surface of the sternum was estimated to be only about 13–19 mm (Halvorsen *et al.*, 1995). Palpation prior to using acupuncture cannot reliably detect the abnormality because tendon fibres, thin connective tissue or bone lamella may conceal the foramen.

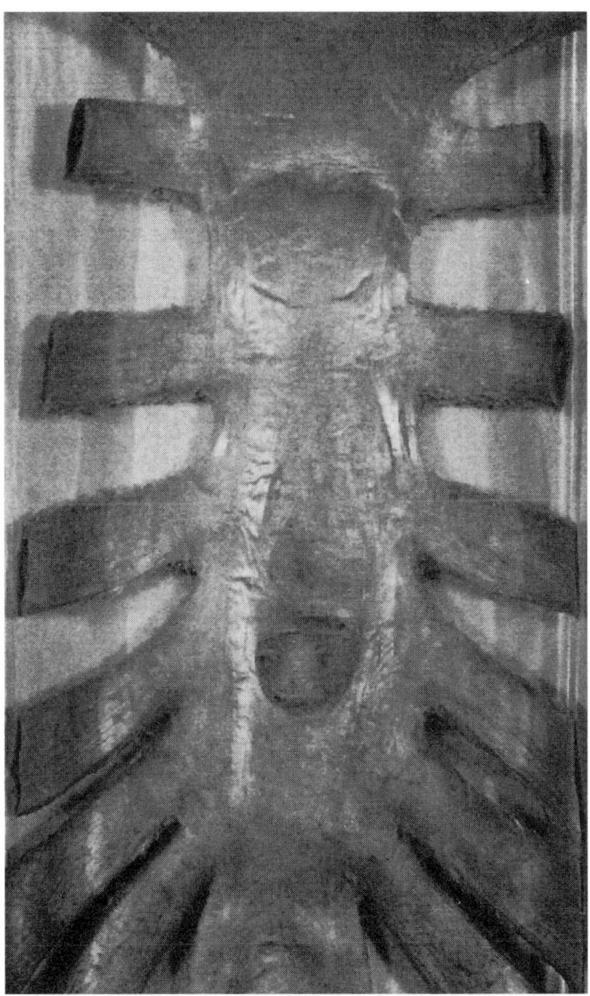

Figure 6.2 Human sternum with foramen sternale; note the superficial covering with bone lamella.

Figure 6.2 shows a human sternum with a foramen sternale covered by a thin bone lamella.

It is clearly impracticable for all patients to undergo CT or MRI before acupuncture. Therefore points over the sternum must be needled tangentially and superficially in order to prevent serious incidents.

Pneumothorax

The most frequently reported injury caused by acupuncture needles is unilateral or bilateral pneumothorax. This chiefly occurs when the needles are placed parasternally or supraclavicularly (Goldberg, 1973; Lewis-Driver, 1973; Fraser, 1974; Waldman, 1974; Stack, 1975; Ritter and Tarala, 1978; Schnorrenberger, 1978; Wex and Weig, 1978; Mazal *et al.*, 1980; Valenta and Hengesh, 1980; Bodner *et al.*, 1983). However, acupuncture to paravertebral, infraclavicular and the lateral thorax regions often causes injuries to the pleurae and lungs (Carron *et al.*, 1974; Kuiper, 1974; Schlenker and Huegel, 1976; Ritter and Tarala, 1978; Wex and Weig, 1978; Mazal *et al.*, 1980; Kropp and Hassler, 1983; Gee, 1984; Willms, 1991; Wright *et al.*, 1991; Vilke and Wulfert, 1997). For further case reports see Smith and Rauscher, 1974; Takishima, 1983; Carette *et al.*, 1984; Henneghien *et al.*, 1984; Schneider and Salzberg, 1984; Gray, 1996; Guerin *et al.*, 1987; Marchuk, 1989; Huet *et al.*, 1990; Morrone *et al.*, 1990; Gray *et al.*, 1991; Marchuk *et al.*, 1993; Despars *et al.*, 1994; Devouassoux *et al.*, 1994; Candela-Blanes *et al.*, 1995; Olusanya and Mansuri, 1997. More than 100 cases of such incidents can be found in scientific publications worldwide, some of which ended fatally (Brettel, 1981; Gee, 1984). In a comprehensive epidemiological survey in Japan, Nakamura *et al.* (1986) examined 664 cases of pneumothorax in women, and came to the conclusion that in 9% of the 255 cases classified as secondary, the cause was acupuncture. In a survey of 1135 doctors and 197 acupuncturists carried out by Norheim and Fønnebø in 1995, 33 cases of pneumothorax were reported. Twenty-one doctors reported 25 cases of pneumothorax and four acupuncturists reported eight cases of pneumothorax. If extrapolated to the whole of the country, this would suggest that 266 cases of acupuncture-induced pneumothorax may have occurred (Norheim and Fønnebø, 1996).

A patient developed symptoms suggestive of pneumothorax following acupuncture. A chest X-ray taken immediately failed to demonstrate the lesion (Ritter and Tarala, 1978). In such cases, it is important to take a repeat X-ray of the patient 24 hours later. The diagnosis of pneumothorax was missed in one case, even though it was evident on X-ray (Wright *et al.*, 1991). Most of the cases reported were admitted and treated with chest drains leading to successful recovery. Haemothorax (Carron *et al.*, 1974) has also been reported but is much rarer. Recent litigation has involved cases of acupuncture-induced pneumothorax (Evans, 1989). One case was settled for 20 000 Australian dollars. Another case involved the failure of a practitioner to diagnose acupuncture-induced pneumothorax. A general practitioner gave acupuncture for frozen shoulder. Needles were inserted in both upper arms of the patient and at the midpoints of both scapulae. Ten minutes later the patient complained of pain and a burning sensation and became short of breath. It was 48 hours later that the condition was diagnosed by another doctor.

There is one case (Waldman, 1974) of a male volunteering to have acupuncture demonstrated at a New Year's party by a man, who proceeded to insert needles in his anterior chest. The volunteer developed chest pain and while in hospital recalled that one needle inserted through his nipple had penetrated his chest much deeper than the other needles. This is clearly a case of malpractice, where the needle was inserted deeply resulting in pneumothorax and in any case the needle was inserted at a site forbidden in traditional acupuncture.

In most of these cases it may be inferred that the therapists did not have a clear understanding of the actual position and borders of the pleurae and lungs, or had insufficient knowledge of the thickness of the soft tissue covering. The most dangerous points – according to the literature – are given in Figure 6.3.

In the supraclavicular region treatment to points stomach (ST) 11 and 12 has caused injuries of the lung; in the infraclavicular region the points lung (LU) 2, ST 13 and kidney (KI) 27 are a potential risk. Furthermore, the parasternal points on the kidney meridian (i.e. KI 22 to KI 27) and the points of the stomach meridian in the midclavicular line (ST 12 to ST 18) need particular caution. Pneumothorax could be easily avoided by good anatomical knowledge and a high degree of caution in the needling of certain points. All practitioners have a responsibility to ensure that they have studied adequately the anatomy of all points at which they propose to insert needles.

From post-mortem examinations, we know that a puncture depth of 10–20 mm, either parasternally or in the region of the midclavicular line,

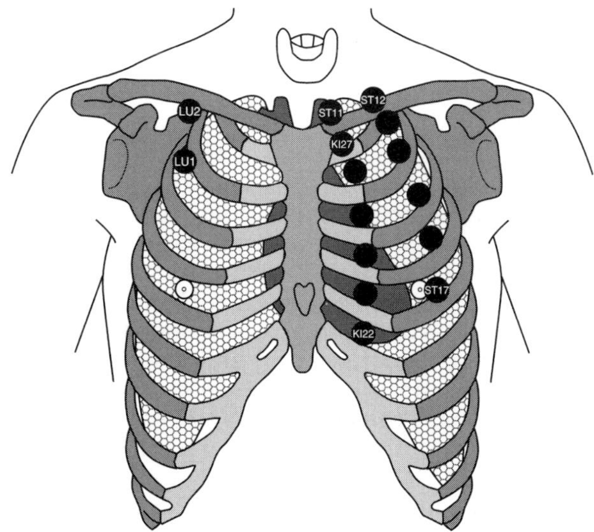

Figure 6.3 Scheme of the chest. ST 11–17, acupuncture points stomach 11–17; KI 22–27, acupuncture points kidney 22–27.

can reach the lungs. It should also be noted that, depending on the thickness of the needle and the amount of tissue resistance, a variable degree of compression of the soft tissue takes place, so that the actual puncturing depth may be considerably greater than the length of the needle. In the region of the lateral branch of the so-called bladder main meridian, which is located approximately in the medial scapular line (acupuncture points bladder (BL) 41 to 54), the surface of the lungs is about 15–20 mm beneath the skin.

Vascular lesions

A common adverse effect is bleeding (Chung, 1980) on withdrawal of the acupuncture needle. This is often minimal and easily dealt with, but rarely can result in bruising at needle sites. In the case of facial acupuncture points, this can result in orbital ecchymosis (Tuke, 1979; Redfearn, 1991). Petechiae (Buchta, 1972) in a child have been reported. A 2-year-old child who was pyrexial and vomiting was seen in accident and emergency in the USA. On examination the child was noted to have multiple petechiae on her back. The clue to the aetiology of the lesions was their symmetrical nature and a history of acupuncture.

Haematoma at the site of needle insertion has been reported (Chung, 1980), possibly due to inadvertent arterial puncture. In this case, a hand was transfixed with one needle using the 'through needle method' to get to LI 4 from small intestine (SI) 3. This resulted in a golf ball sized haematoma. A case of pseudoaneurysm probably caused by acupuncture was reported in 1994 (Fujiwara *et al.*, 1994). A woman had been treated for shoulder stiffness several times with 20–30 needles around the spines of the scapulae each session. After the fourth session she noticed a nodule at her left shoulder and experienced a sharp pain. After diagnosis with CT and angiography, surgery was performed and a partially thrombosed pseudoaneurysm in the region of the costocervical artery was found. Another case of an aneurysm due to acupuncture was reported in 1996 (Lord and Schwartz, 1996). Deep puncturing of the point BL 40 caused a lesion of the posterior wall of the popliteal artery which led to a false aneurysm. Figure 6.4 shows the close relationship between the incriminated point and the popliteal vessels.

A compartment syndrome has been reported (Smith *et al.*, 1989) following acupuncture in an anticoagulated patient. A 68-year-old man who was taking warfarin because he had a prosthetic heart valve, had received acupuncture from a physician. One of the needles was inserted at ST 36. Almost immediately, the patient developed local pain that worsened. There was gradual swelling and discoloration over 4 days resulting in hospital admission. An anterior compartment surgical decompression fasciotomy was carried out. It is not clear whether the acupuncturist was aware of the patient's medical history and current medication.

There have been two reports (Ruchkin, 1987; Blanchard, 1991) of deep venous thrombophlebitis following acupuncture. Another case (Gray, 1996) mimicking a deep venous thrombosis was a 72-year-old female with rheumatoid arthritis, who had acupuncture around her right knee.

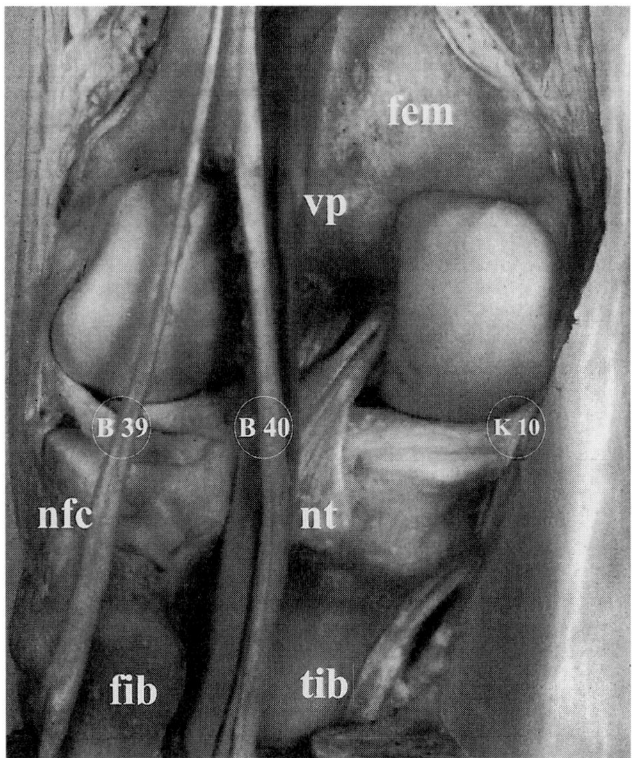

Figure 6.4 Left fossa poplitea. BL 39/40, acupuncture points bladder 39/40. fem = femur; fib = fibula; nfc = nervus fibularis communis; nt = nervus tibialis; tib = tibia; vp = vasa poplitea.

One week later she returned with pain in the back of her knee and ankle swelling. Her practitioner arranged an urgent referral to the local hospital, where she was commenced on anticoagulants. However, a venogram carried out later was normal and it was concluded that a Baker's cyst had burst.

It is likely that the rate of more or less severe lesions of peripheral vessels resulting from acupuncture which are undetected and unpublished may be rather high.

Trauma to spinal cord

There have been a number of reports, mainly from Japan, of trauma to the spinal cord and spinal nerve roots during needle insertion (Noumi *et al.*, 1976; Kondo *et al.*, 1979; Shiraishi *et al.*, 1979; Sasaki *et al.*, 1984; Tomonaga *et al.*, 1984; Isu *et al.*, 1985; Kojima *et al.*, 1985; Maruoka *et al.*, 1986; Kida *et al.*, 1988; Hasegawa *et al.*, 1990; Kishikawa *et al.*, 1990; Sato *et al.*, 1991; Matsui *et al.*, 1992) or caused by the migration of cut or broken retained needles (Drake, 1974). Trauma to the patient (e.g. a fall) can result in movement of a retained needle, leading to injury of vital structures. Patients present with focal neurological signs and radiological examinations reveal the retained needles, which then require surgical removal. The level of the lesion varied from C1/2 to S1. The distance from the surface of the skin to the spinal cord or the roots of the spinal nerves ranges from 25 to 45 mm when inserting a needle in the paravertebral line, depending on the constitution of the patient. Deep needling of points of the inner branch of the bladder meridian (BL 11 to BL 20) and the governing vessel (GV) (Figure 6.5) was particularly likely to cause lesions of the spinal cord or the spinal nerve roots.

There have been isolated reports of spinal arachnoiditis (Oka *et al.*, 1986) and subarachnoid haemorrhage (Murata *et al.*, 1990; Keane *et al.*, 1993). Nerve injury resulting in sympathetic dystrophy has been reported (Kataoka and Sakata, 1958; Carron *et al.*, 1974).

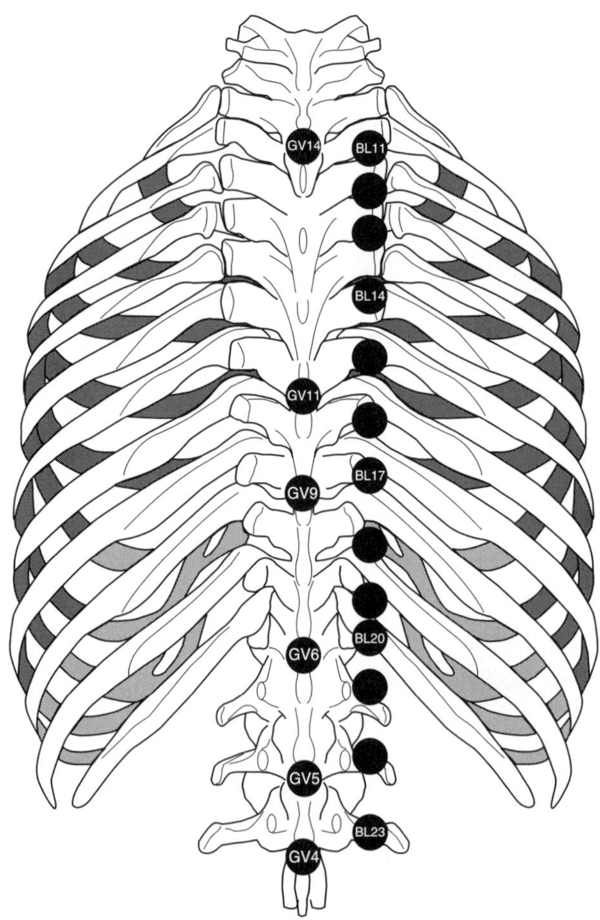

Figure 6.5 Scheme of the spine. BL 11–23, acupuncture points bladder 11–23; GV 4–14, acupuncture points governing vessel 4–14.

Trauma to peripheral nerves

Injuries of peripheral nerves are reported less frequently. Two published case reports have been found which clearly relate to acupuncture. In one case a broken needle in the carpal tunnel caused a neuropathy of the median nerve (Southworth and Hartwig, 1990). This nerve can be damaged by needling the points CV 6 and CV 7 and in the case of a slightly atypical course, even by puncturing LU 8. In the other case, a needle that was inserted in the region of the fibular head led to a complete paralysis of the fibular nerve and foot-drop (Sobel *et al.*, 1997). The fibular nerve is particularly variable in its course. Figure 6.4 illustrates the back of a left knee. The close topographical relationship of the points BL 39 and BL 40 to the fibular and tibial nerve is demonstrated. Figure 6.6 shows the lateral view on another knee.

A relatively high course of the fibular nerve close to the point gall bladder (GB) 34 can be noted. One may safely assume that the number of

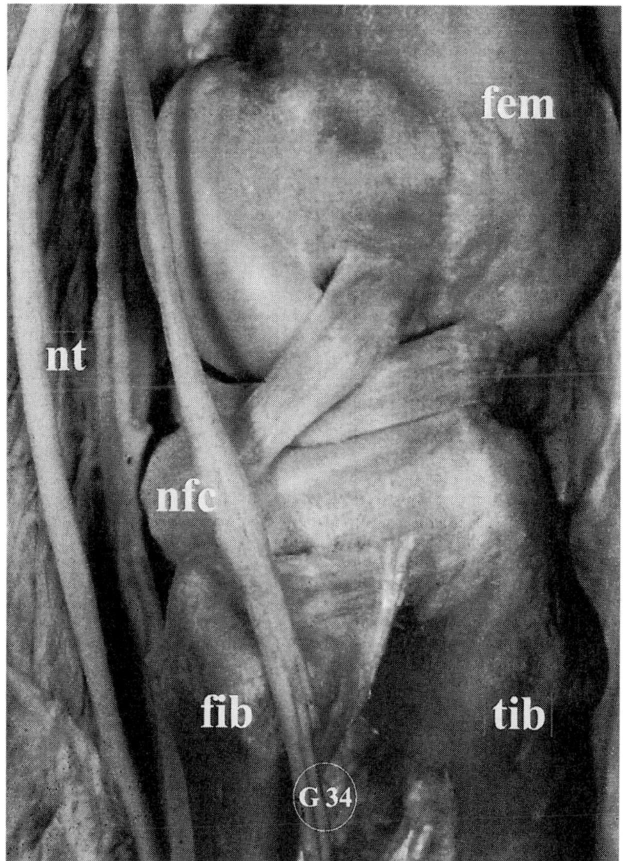

Figure 6.6 Right knee from lateral. fem = femur; fib = fibula; nfc = nervus fibularis communis; nt = nervus tibialis; tib = tibia.

undetected cases of transient or persistent nerve injuries due to acupuncture is much higher than the number of the reported cases.

Lesions in the skin

It is not uncommon to observe transient erythema at needle sites. This is most likely caused by local histamine release from skin trauma. Patients with an atopic tendency are more likely to develop transient erythema at the needle site (Bodnar, 1965; Dung, 1987).

There have been reports of contact dermatitis (Castelain *et al.*, 1987) to nickel (Fisher, 1976; Romaguera and Grimalt, 1979, 1981), chromium (Tanii *et al.*, 1991) and zinc (Koizumi *et al.*, 1989). All cases were reported in individuals who had a history of allergy and had positive patch tests for the respective metals. Some workers have linked acupuncture with various dermatological oddities such as prurigo pigmentosa (Tanii *et al.*, 1991), blue macules of localized argyria (Tanita *et al.*, 1985), a case of multiple lymphocytoma cutis of the ears (Bork, 1983) and even a case of skin carcinoma (Tsukerman, 1970). The latter was one of the more speculative case reports and was published in Russian with an English abstract. Koebner phenomena at the needle insertion sites has been described in a patient suffering from psoriasis (Kirschbaum, 1972). A case of abrasions of the shoulder (Carron *et al.*, 1974) has been reported, where a sharp instrument was used to abrade skin in addition to needle insertion. Localized lipoatrophy after acupuncture has been reported in two patients (Drago *et al.*, 1996). Both female patients developed symmetrical symptomless depressions on the lateral aspect of their arms. These lesions developed 3 months after acupuncture treatment. Biopsy revealed characteristic histopathological changes seen in involutional lipoatrophy.

A case (Chang, 1974) of reactivation of cutaneous herpetic lesions following 12 hours after each acupuncture treatment has been reported. A 67-year-old female with cutaneous herpes had 15 recurrences after 20 acupuncture treatments over a 5-month period. The lesions occurred at the same site, which was distant from the needle site.

Moxibustion

In China and the Far East, acupuncture has been combined with other therapeutic modalities such as herbs, massage and moxibustion. Moxa is the dried leaves of *Artemisia vulgaris* made into various forms: 'punk' is loose moxa, rather like green cotton wool, while 'moxa-rolls' are like cigars. When lit, moxa smoulders constantly. The heat is usually applied gently by holding a glowing moxa-roll about 2 cm from the point. Carelessness in the technique can result in accidental burns. However, in the Far East 'cauterizing moxibustion' is often used, where cones of loose punk are burned intentionally on the skin until blisters form. Third degree burns, eschars and scars (Carron *et al.*, 1974) have been reported from the use of moxibustion. Hot needle acupuncture, which entails inserting a heated needle, has also resulted in scarring (Hung and Mines, 1991). Inhalations of moxa fumes during treatment resulted in a practitioner developing chest tightness, dyspnoea and mucus production (Umeh, 1989). The practitioner had a tendency to asthma and bronchitis. Antihistamine prophylaxis minimized such attacks, confirming an allergic origin to the symptoms.

Miscellaneous

Electroacupuncture

This can impair the function of a demand type pacemaker (Fujiwara *et al.*, 1980). Low-frequency electroacupuncture employed for anaesthesia during a cervical operation deranged the proper function of a demand pacemaker. An applied voltage of about 20 V and a current of about 3 mA resulted in complete inhibition of the pacemaker. It would be prudent not to administer electroacupuncture to any patient with a pacemaker.

Retained needles

There have been reports of acupuncture needles in the abdominal cavity (Yin, 1937), kidney parenchyma (Fukuda *et al.*, 1969; Yamaguchi *et al.*, 1989) and the urinary tract, leading to calculus formation (Keller *et al.*, 1972; Aso et al, 1979; Yuzawa *et al.*, 1991). A man presented with haematuria and an X-ray revealed a metallic object in his pelvis. An acupuncture needle was retrieved by cystoscopy. He admitted inserting the needle into the urethral meatus to clear some glue which had become stuck to his penis (Roy, 1974). Foreign-body granuloma reaction to retained acupuncture needles has been noted (Asano, 1969; Chun and Cho, 1991). There have been reports (Behrstock and Petrakis, 1974; Imray and Hiramatsu, 1975; Saenz *et al.*, 1978; Campbell, 1982; Galuten and Austin, 1988; Hollander *et al.*, 1991; Gerard *et al.*, 1993) of fine linear metallic foreign bodies found incidentally on various X-rays. The patients, usually of oriental origin, give a history of having had acupuncture by the okibari technique. This is a controversial technique peculiar to Japan, where gold needles are inserted into the skin permanently, the protruding part being cut off. The number of permanent subcutaneous needles varies widely; one patient had over 200 needles. A recent case (Chiu and Austin, 1995) involved a 42-year-old Japanese male whose X-rays revealed many fine metallic opacities in the soft tissues of his back. Needles do occasionally break off accidentally (Rogers, 1981) while in use. This is often due to muscle movement or spasm during treatment and is more likely to occur if old needles are being used. Patients should be advised not to move during treatment and the condition of the needles checked when they are removed. If breakage has occurred, the fragments must be removed immediately. The practitioner must remember to remove all inserted needles.

Other

A 29-year-old man was found to have increased bone activity on bone scans (Kuno and Cerqueira, 1995). He had a bone scan (scintigraphy with

^{99m}Tc-methylene diphosphonate) for the investigation of chronic back pain. Posterior and lateral images of the skull showed focal increased uptake in several regions of his skull. On further questioning, he related that he had received acupuncture for his condition at the same regions as the increased uptake. The needle sites were confirmed by the patient's acupuncturist. The authors of the report suggest that acupuncture be added as yet another cause for increased activity on bone scans.

Conclusions

The majority of the case reports of adverse effects of acupuncture did not have sufficient information to critically appraise them. Future case reports of adverse reactions should give details about the type of acupuncture involved, who gave it, the timing of the adverse reaction, its reversibility and any confounding factors. All future clinical trials involving acupuncture should prospectively identify adverse effects, a good example being the study by Kelleher *et al.* (1994). At present the information on the incidence and prevalence of adverse effects of acupuncture is poorly described in the literature. Previous surveys with differing methodologies indicate that there is a significant but low risk of serious side-effects of acupuncture from 1 : 10 000 to 1 : 100 000 (White *et al.* 1997). Umlauf recorded 14 340 patients who received 139 988 acupuncture treatments at the Brno-Bohuncie Hospital in Czechoslovakia between 1975 and 1985 (Umlauf, 1988). The main indications for treatment were painful disorders. Umlauf noted a total of 8.9% of patients experienced adverse effects (syncope, haematoma, pneumothorax and retained needles). In a questionnaire sent to 1135 doctors and 197 acupuncturists in Norway (Norheim and Fønnebø, 1996) enquiring about adverse effects of acupuncture, 12% of doctors and 31% of acupuncturists reported adverse effects of acupuncture. In a survey of readers of the British daily newspaper, *The Guardian*, 386 people responded to an invitation to answer a questionnaire about their use of complementary therapies (Abbott *et al.*, 1996). Experiencing adverse effects following acupuncture was reported by 12.5%. A survey of general practitioners in Devon and Cornwall enquiring whether they had encountered patients experiencing adverse reactions due to complementary therapies elicited more serious adverse reactions than those reported by the users in *The Guardian* survey.

Nearly 4000 acupuncture practitioners were registered members of UK professional acupuncture bodies in 1997 (Mills and Peacock, 1997). There may be an equal number who were not registered. In Germany, it is estimated that more than 20 000 practitioners carry out therapy by means of acupuncture. In 1997 there were about 8700 licensed acupuncturists in the USA. Three per cent of the adult population of the UK alone consulted acupuncturists in 1984 (Fulder, 1988). It has been calculated that more than 10 million acupuncture treatments are given in the USA every year (Marwick, 1997). These figures suggest a very low prevalence of adverse reactions. It is likely that the rate of more or less severe incidents due to acupuncture which are undetected and unpublished may be rather high. In response to the paucity of information on the epidemiology of adverse effects of acupuncture, the Department of Complementary Medicine at Exeter University (UK) is co-ordinating a prospective survey of 30 000 acupuncture treatments (White *et al.*, 1997). This major undertaking aims to accurately assess the risk of adverse effects of acupuncture.

Ancient practitioners of acupuncture were aware of adverse effects and the 'Nei-Jing' lists contraindications. For example, 'if the patient has come from far away, treatment should be given in a lying position after the patient has taken a good rest'. This is a sensible precaution. However, there are other more controversial recommendations such as 'needling is forbidden after sexual intercourse, and sexual intercourse should be avoided after needling' (Luwen, 1990). We make the following recommendations based upon the results of our review of the scientific literature (Table 6.1).

The serious adverse effects reported in the literature may easily be prevented by straightforward precautions. Some of the adverse effects were due to unusual or even controversial forms of acupuncture.

In most countries the control of training programmes in acupuncture is insufficient (Ernst and White, 1997a). Quality standards (if they exist at all) are set by the individual professional bodies, which are often commercially orientated. Many medical practitioners commence training in acupuncture after they have been practising in their profession for some time without the need for profound anatomical knowledge (Peuker and Filler, 1997b). The anatomical and medical knowledge of non-medically qualified practitioners needs to be of a sufficient level in order to ensure the safety of the patient. The above evidence implies that this can cause irreparable damage to patients. There is a need for practitioners and patients to be aware of possible adverse effects of acupuncture, the majority of which can be avoided with cautious and prudent use of this ancient therapy.

Table 6.1 Cases in which acupuncture is contraindicated

Patients taking anticoagulant medication
Press needles in patients with prosthetic or damaged heart valves
Electroacupuncture in patients with pacemaker
Particular caution required:
Acupuncture points on thorax
Immunosuppressed patients
General precautions always necessary:
Remember orthodox diagnostic skills
Use sterile disposable needles
Use aseptic technique with press needles
Lie the patient down during treatment
Advise patient to avoid driving after treatment
Count needles before and after treatment
Observe patient for bleeding

Adapted from Box 19.1 in Rampes 1998.

References

Abbot, N., White, A. R. and Ernst, E. (1996). Complementary medicine. *Nature,* **381,** 361.

Alexander, P., Hamilton-Fairly, G. and Smithers, D. W. (1974). Repeated acupuncture and serum hepatitis. *Br. Med. J.,* **271,** 46.

Alexis, J., Lubin, J. and Bichachi, A. (1988). Acupuncture and non-A, non-B hepatitis. *South. Med. J.,* **81,** 101.

Allison, G. and Kravitz, E. (1975). Auricular chondritis secondary to acupuncture. *N. Engl. J. Med.,* **293,** 780.

Asano, K. (1969). Foreign body granuloma caused by a broken sitren needle for acupuncture. *Otolaryngology (Tokyo),* **41,** 289–291.

Aso, Y., Murahashi, I. and Yokoyama, M. (1979). Foreign body stone of the ureter as a complication of acupuncture. *Eur. Urol.,* **5,** 57–59.

Baltimore, R. S. and Moloy, P. J. (1976). Perichondritis of the ear as a complication of acupuncture. *Arch. Otolaryngol.,* **102,** 572–573.

Batisse, C. (1986). Acupuncture followed by hepatitis. *Rev. Rhum. Mal. Osteoartic.,* **53,** 670.

Behrstock, B. B. and Petrakis, N. L. (1974). Permanent subcutaneous gold acupuncture needles. *West. J. Med.,* **121,** 140–142.

Blanchard, B. M. (1991). Deep vein thrombophlebitis after acupuncture. *Ann. Intern. Med.,* **115,** 748.

Bodnar, P. N. (1965). On the eosinopenic reaction to acupuncture in patients with bronchial asthma. *Vrach. Delo,* **9,** 147.

Bodner, G., Topilsky, M. and Grief, J. (1983). Pneumothorax as a complication of acupuncture in the treatment of bronchial asthma. *Ann. Allergy,* **51,** 401–403.

Bork, K. (1983). Multiple lymphocytoma at the point of puncture as complication of acupuncture treatment. Traumatic origin of lymphocytoma. *Hautarzt,* **34,** 496–499.

Bostrom, H. and Rossner, S. (1990). Quality of alternative medicine – complications and avoidable deaths. *Qual. Assur. Health Care,* **2,** 11–17.

Boxall, E. H. (1978). Acupuncture hepatitis in the West Midlands, 1977. *J. Med. Virol.,* **2,** 377–379.

Brattberg, G. (1986). Acupuncture treatments: a traffic hazard? *Am. J. Acupunct.,* **14,** 265–267.

Brettel, H. (1981). Akupunktur als Todesursache. *MMWR,* **123,** 97–98.

Brougham, P.A. (1988). Case reports. An interesting acupuncture phenomenon. *Acupunct. Med.,* **5,** 9.

Buchta, R. M. (1972). An unusual cause of petechiae. *Am. J. Dis. Child.,* **123,** 613.

Buck, C. C. (1986). Propagated needle sensation. *J. Chin. Med.,* **22,** 15–16.

Campbell, A. E. R. (1982). Hazards of acupuncture. *Br. J. Radiol.,* **55,** 875–877.

Candela-Blanes, A., Hernandez-Blasco, L., Martin-Serrano, C. and Romero-Candeira, S. (1995). Pneumothorax as a complication of acupuncture. *Ann. Med. Interne,* **12,** 412–413.

Carette, M. F., Mayaud, C., Houacine, S. *et al.* (1984). Acupuncture treatment of acute asthma: probable role in the onset of pneumothorax with progression to a state of status asthmaticus. *Rev. Pneumol. Clin.,* **40,** 69–70.

Carron, H., Epstein, B. S. and Grand, B. (1974). Complications of acupuncture. *JAMA,* **228,** 1552–1554.

Castelain, M., Castelain, P. Y. and Ricciardi, R. (1987). Contact dermatitis to acupuncture needles. *Contact Dermatitis,* **16,** 44.

Castro, K. G., Lifson, A. R., White, C. R. *et al.* (1988). Investigations of AIDS patients with no previously identified risk factors. *JAMA,* **259,** 1338–1342.

Chamberland, M. E., Conley, L. J. and Buehler, J. W. (1989). Unusual modes of HIV transmission. *N. Engl. J. Med.,* **321,** 1476.

Chang, T. W. (1974). Activation of cutaneous herpes by acupuncture. *N. Engl. J. Med.,* **290,** 1310.

Chen, C. Y., Liu, G. C., Sheu, R. S. and Huang, C. L. (1997). Bacterial meningitis and lumbar epidural hematoma due to lumbar acupunctures: a case report. *Kao Hsiung I Hsueh Ko Hsueh Tsa Chih,* **13,** 328–331.

Chen, F., Hwang, S., Lee, H. *et al.* (1990). Clinical study of syncope during acupuncture treatment. *Acupunct. Electrother. Res.*, **15,** 107–119.
Cheng, T. O. (1983). Acupuncture needles as a cause of bacterial endocarditis. *Br. Med.J.*, **287,** 689.
Cheng, T. O. (1991). Pericardial effusion from self inserted needle in the heart. *Eur. Heart J.*, **12,** 958.
Chiu, E. S. and Austin, J. H. M. (1995). Acupuncture needle fragments. *N. Engl. J. Med.*, **332,** 304.
Chun, S. I. and Cho, S. W. (1991). Silica granuloma: scanning electron microscopy and energy dispersive X-ray microanalysis. *J. Dermatol.*, **18,** 92–96.
Chung, C. (1980). Common errors and complications in acupuncture treatment. *Acupunct. Res. Q.*, **4,** 51–58.
Communicable Diseases Surveillance Centre of the PHLS. (1977). Acupuncture associated hepatitis in the West Midlands in 1977. *Br. Med. J.*, **2,** 1610.
Communicable Diseases Surveillance Centre of the PHLS. (1992). Hepatitis B associated with an acupuncture clinic. *Communicable Disease Rep. Weekly*, **2**(48). 27 November.
Conn, H. (1988). Acupuncture in epidemic HBV hepatitis: in China too? *Hepatology*, **8,** 1176–1177.
Cooper, P., Stewart, J. and McCormick, W. (1988). Development and morphology of the sternal foramen. *Am. J. Forensic Med. Pathol.*, **9,** 342–347.
Corbett, M. and Sinclair, M. (1974). Acu and pleuro–puncture. *N. Engl. J. Med.*, **290,** 167–168.
Davis, O. and Powell, W. (1985). Auricular perichondritis secondary to acupuncture. *Arch. Otolaryngol.*, **111,** 770–771.
De Galocsy, C., Geubel, A. P., Gulbis, A. and Dive, C. (1982). Hepatite sur acupuncture: Rapport de sept cas. *Acta Gastroenterol. Belg.*, **45,** 224–230.
Despars, J., Sassoon, C. and Light, R. (1994). Significance of iatrogenic pneumothoraces. *Chest*, **105,** 1147–1150.
Devouassoux, G., Kelkel, E. and Delormas, P. (1994). Bilateral pneumothorax with an unusual origin. *Rev. Pneumol. Clin.*, **50,** 186–187.
Dominguez, A., Milicua, J. M., Larraona, J. L. *et al.* (1985). Viral hepatitis B transmitted by acupuncture: presentation of 5 cases. *Med. Clin. (Barc.)*, **84,** 317–319.
Doutsu, Y., Tao, Y., Sasayama, K. *et al.* (1986). A case of *Staphylococcus aureus* septicemia after acupuncture therapy. *Kansenshogaku Zasshi*, **60,** 911–916.
Drago, F., Rongioletti, F., Battifoglio, M. L. and Rebora, A. (1996). Localised lipoatrophy after acupuncture. *Lancet*, **347,** 1484.
Drake, T. E. (1974). Complication of acupuncture. *JAMA*, **229,** 1285–1286.
Dung, H. C. (1987). An immediate atopic erythroid reaction induced by acupuncture needles on the posterior thoracic wall. *Altern. Med.*, **2,** 209–214.
Eisenberg, D. M., Kessler, R. C., Foster, C. *et al.* (1993). Unconventional medicine in the United States: prevalence, costs and patterns of use. *N. Engl. J. Med.*, **328,** 246–252.
Ernst, E. (1995). The risks of acupuncture. *Int. J. Risk Saf. Med.*, **6,** 179–186.
Ernst, E. and White, A. (1997a). Acupuncture: safety first. *Br. Med. J.*, **314,** 1362.
Ernst, E. and White, A. (1997b). Life-threatening adverse reactions of acupuncture? A systematic review. *Pain*, **71,** 123–126.
Evans, M. (1989). Litigation and ethical issues affecting acupuncture. *Acupunct. Med.*, **6,** 24–27.
Fisher, A. A. (1976). Allergic dermatitis from acupuncture needles. *Cutis*, **38,** 226.
Fraser, R. M (1974). An unusual complication of acupuncture. *Can. Med. Assoc. J.*, **3,** 388–393.
Fujiwara, H., Taniguchi, K., Takeuchi, J. and Ikezono, E. (1980). The influence of low frequency acupuncture on a demand pacemaker. *Chest*, **78,** 1285–1286.
Fujiwara, T., Tanohata, K. and Nagase, M. (1994). Pseudoaneurysm caused by acupuncture: a rare complication. *AJR*, **162,** 731.
Fukuda, K., Kiriyama, T., Kashawagi, T. *et al.* (1969). Foreign bodies (acupuncture needles) in kidney combined with a stone. *Acta Urol. Japon. (Kyoto)*, **15,** 233–236.

Fulder, S. (1988). *The Handbook of Complementary Medicine*, chap. 2:28. New York, Oxford: University Press.

Galuten, A. and Austin, J. H. M. (1988). Permanent subcutaneous acupuncture needles: radiographic manifestations. *J. Can. Radiol. Assoc.*, **39,** 54–56.

Garcia-Bengoechea, M., Cabriada, J., Arriola, J. A. and Arenas, J. I. (1985). Hepatitis B caused by acupuncture and the same acupuncturist. *Med. Clin. Barc.*, **85,** 686.

Gee, D. (1984). Fatal pneumothorax due to acupuncture. *Br. Med. J.*, **288,** 114.

Gerard, P. S., Wilck, E. and Schiano, T. (1993). Imaging implications in the evaluation of permanent needle acupuncture. *Clin. Imaging*, **17,** 36–40.

Gilbert, J. G. (1987). Auricular complications of acupuncture. *N. Z. Med. J.*, **100,** 141–142.

Goldberg, I. (1973). Pneumothorax associated with acupuncture. *Med. J. Aust.*, **1,** 941–942.

Gray, P. (1996). Baker's cyst burst after acupuncture. *Acupunct. Med.*, **14**(1), 41–42.

Gray, R., Maharajh, G. S. and Hyland, R. (1991). Pneumothorax resulting from acupuncture. *Can. Assoc. Radiol. J.*, **42**(2), 139–140.

Guerin, J. M., Tibourtine, O., Lhote, F. and Segrestaa, J. M. (1987). 2 cases of pneumothorax following acupuncture. *Rev. Med. Interne*, **8**(1), 71.

HMSO (1986). *AIDS: Don't Die of Ignorance*. DHSS leaflet. London: HMSO.

HMSO (1989). Guidelines for the Blood Transfusion Services in the United Kingdom, vol. 1, chap. 5:22. London: HMSO.

Hadden, W. A. and Swanson. A. J. G. (1982). Spinal infection caused by acupuncture mimicking a prolapsed intervertebral disc. *J. Bone Joint Surg.*, **64A,** 624–626.

Halvorsen, T. B., Anda, S. S., Naess, A. B. and Levang, O. W. (1995). Fatal cardiac tamponade after acupuncture through congenital sternal foramen. *Lancet*, **345,** 1175.

Harada, K., Suzuki, T., Suzuki, A. *et al.* (1997). Toxic shock-like syndrome after acupuncturation. *Kansenshogaku Zasshi*, **71,** 1066–1070.

Hasegawa, O., Shibuya, K., Suzuki, Y. and Nagatomo, H. (1990). Acupuncture needles, straying in the central nervous system and presenting neurological signs and symptoms. *Rinsho Shinkeigaku*, **30,** 1109–1113.

Hasegawa, J., Noguchi, N., Yamasaki, J. *et al.* (1991). Delayed cardiac tamponade and hemothorax induced by an acupuncture needle. *Cardiology*, **78,** 58–63.

Hayhoe, S. and Pitt, E. (1987). Case reports. Complications of acupuncture. *Acupunct. Med.*, **4,** 15.

Henneghien, C., Bruart, J. and Remacle, P. (1984). A new iatrogenic pathology: pneumothorax after acupuncture. *Rev. Pneumol. Clin.*, **40,** 197–199.

Hollander, J. E., Dewitz, A. and Bowers, S. (1991). Permanently imbedded subcutaneous acupuncture needles: radiographic appearance. *Ann. Emerg. Med.*, **20,** 1025–1026.

Huet, R., Renard, E., Blotman, M. J. and Jaffiol, C. (1990). Unrecognised pneumothorax after acupuncture in a female patient with anorexia nervosa. *Presse Med*, **19,** 1415.

Hung, V. C. and Mines, J. S. (1991). Eschars and scarring from hot needle acupuncture treatment. *J. Am. Acad. Dermatol.*, **24,** 148–149.

Hussain, K. K. (1974). Serum hepatitis associated with repeated acupuncture. *Br. Med. J.*, **3,** 41–42.

Imray, T. J. and Hiramatsu, Y. (1975). Radiographic manifestations of Japanese acupuncture. *Radiology*, **115,** 625–626.

Isu, T., Iwasaki, Y., Sasaki, H. and Abe, H. (1985). Spinal cord and root injuries due to glass fragments and acupuncture needles. *Surg. Neurol.*, **23,** 255–260.

Izatt, E. and Fairman, M. (1977). Staphylococcal septicaemia with DIC associated with acupuncture. *Postgrad. Med. J.*, **53,** 285–286.

Jefferys, D. B., Smith, S., Brennand-Roper, D. A. and Curry, P. V. L. (1983). Acupuncture needles as a cause of bacterial endocarditis. *Br. Med. J.*, **287,** 326–327.

Johansen, M. and Nielsen, K. O. (1990). Perichondritis of the ear caused by acupuncture. *Ugeskr. Laeger*, **152,** 172–173.

Jones, R. O. and Cross, G. (1980). Suspected chronic osteomyelitis secondary to acupuncture treatment. *J. Am. Podiatr. Med. Assoc.*, **70,** 149–151.

Kataoka, H. and Sakata, M. (1958). Nerve injury due to an acupuncture treatment. *Geka*, **20,** 578–582.

Kataoka, H. J. (1997). Cardiac tamponade caused by penetration of an acupuncture needle into the right ventricle. *Thorac. Cardiovasc. Surg.*, **14,** 674–676.

Keane, J. R., Ahmadi, J. and Gruen, P. (1993). Spinal epidural hematoma with subarachnoid hemorrhage caused by acupuncture. *Am. J. Neuroradiol.*, **14,** 365–366.

Kelleher, C. J., Filshie, J., Burton, G. *et al.* (1994). Acupuncture and the treatment of irritative bladder symptoms. *Acupunct. Med.*, **12,** 9–12.

Keller, W .J., Parker, S. G. and Garvin, J. P. (1972). Possible renal complications of acupuncture. *JAMA*, **222,** 1559.

Kent, G. P., Brondum, J., Keenlyside, R. A. *et al.* (1988). A large outbreak of acupuncture associated hepatitis B. *Am. J. Epidemiol.*, **127,** 591–598.

Kida, Y., Naritomi, H., Sawada, T. *et al.* (1988). Cervical spinal cord injury caused by acupuncture. *Arch. Neurol.*, **45,** 831.

Kirschbaum, J. O. (1972). Koebner phenomenon following acupuncture. *Arch Dermatol.*, **106,** 767.

Kirschenbaum, A. E. and Rizzo, C. (1997). Glenohumeral pyarthrosis following acupuncture treatment. *Orthopedics*, **20,** 1184–1186.

Kishikawa, K., Nakae, Y., Fujiwara, S. *et al.* (1990). A spinal cord injury caused by acupuncture needles. *Pain Clin.*, **3,** 179–184.

Kiyosawa, K., Gibo, Y., Sodeyama, T. *et al.* (1987). Possible infectious causes in 651 patients with acute viral hepatitis during a 10-year period (1976–1985). *Liver*, **7,** 163–168.

Kobler, E., Schmuzigar, P. and Harmann, G. (1979). Hepatitis nach Akupunktur. *Schweiz. Med. Wochenschr.*, **109,** 1828–1829.

Koizumi, H., Tomoyori, T., Kumakri, M. and Ohkawara, A. (1989). Acupuncture needle dermatitis. *Contact Dermatitis*, **21,** 352.

Kojima, Y., Ono, K., Ogino, H. *et al.* (1985). Migration of the needle of acupuncture into the cervical spinal canal. Report of four cases. *Chuba Nippon Seikeigeka Gakkai Zasshi*, **23,** 292–294.

Kondo, A., Koyama, T., Ishikawa, J. and Yamasaki, T. (1979). Injury to the spinal cord produced by acupuncture needle. *Surg. Neurol.*, **11,** 155–156.

Kropp, R. and Hassler, R. (1983). Accidental pneumothorax following injections and acupuncture in the thoracic region. *Med. Welt.*, **34,** 1143–1144.

Kuiper, J. J. (1974). Pneumothorax as complication of acupuncture. *JAMA*, **229**, 1422.

Kuno, R.C. and Cerqueira, M.D. (1995). Enhanced bone metabolism induced by acupuncture. *J. Nucl. Med.*, **36,** 2246–2247.

Lapeer, G. and Monga, T. N. (1988). Pain secondary to acupuncture therapy. *Cranio*, **6,** 188–190.

Lee, R. J. and Mcilwain, J. C. (1985). Subacute bacterial endocarditis following ear acupuncture. *Int. J. Cardiol.*, **7,** 62–63.

Lewis-Driver, D. J. (1973). Pneumothorax associated with acupuncture. *Med. J. Aust.*, **2,** 296.

Li, F. P. and Shiang, E. (1980). Acupuncture and possible hepatitis B infection. *JAMA*, **243,** 1423.

Lord, R. and Schwartz, P. (1996). False aneurysm of the popliteal artery complicating acupuncture. *Aust. N. Z. Surg.*, **66,** 645–647.

Luwen, G. (1990). Understanding the theory of acupuncture contra-indications according to the Nei Jing. *J. Chin. Med.*, **34,** 31–32.

Marchuk, I. K. (1989). Pneumothorax developing as a result of acupuncture in the treatment of bronchial asthma. *Vrach. Delo*, **5,** 101–102.

Marchuk, I., Kuz'mich, V., Marchuk, L. and Ordynskii, N. (1993). Iatrogenic pneumothorax. *Lik Sprava*, **10–12**, 81–82.

Maruoka, N., Kinoshita, K. and Wakisaka, S. (1986). Cervical spinal cord injury caused by a broken acupuncture needle: a case report. *No Shinkei Geka*, **14,** 785–787.

Marwick, C. (1997). Acceptance of some acupuncture applications. *JAMA*, **278,** 1725–1727.

Matsui, S., Matsuoka, K., Nakagawa, K. *et al.* (1992). Cervical spinal cord injury caused by a broken acupuncture needle: a case report. *No Shinkei Geka*, **20,** 499–503.

Mazal, D. A., King, T., Harvey, J. and Cohen, J. (1980). Bilateral pneumothorax after acupuncture. *N. Engl. J. Med.*, **302,** 1365–1366.

Mills, S. and Peacock, W. (1997). Professional Organisation of Complementary and Alternative Medicine in the United Kingdom: A Report to the Department of Health. Exeter: Centre for Complementary Health Studies.

Moro-Aguado, J., De-la-Lama-Lopez-Areal, J. and Cortejoso-Gonzalo, B. (1985). Viral hepatitis B transmitted by acupucture. *Med. Clin. Barc.*, **85,** 344.

Morrone, N., Freire, J. A., Ferreira, A. K. and Dourado, A. M. (1990). Iatrogenic pneumothorax caused by acupuncture. *Rev. Paul. Med.*, **108,** 189–191.

Murata, K., Nishio, A., Nishikawa, M. *et al.* (1990). Subarachnoid hemorrhage and spinal root injury caused by acupuncture needle. *Neurol. Med. Chir. (Tokyo)*, **30,** 956–959.

Nakamura, H., Konishiike, J., Sugamura, A. and Takeno, Y. (1986). Epidemiology of spontaneous pneumothorax in women. *Chest*, **89,** 378–382.

Negro, F. E., Bornoroni, C. and Bove, G. (1977). Complications in acupuncture: viral hepatitis. *Minn. Med.*, **68,** 727–728.

Nieda, S., Abe, T., Kuribayashi, R. *et al.* (1973). Cardiac trauma as complication of acupuncture treatment: a case report of cardiac tamponade resulting from a broken needle. *Jpn. J. Thorac. Surg.*, **293,** 780.

Norheim, A. J. and Fønnebø, V. (1996). Adverse effects are more than occasional case reports: results from questionnaires among 1135 randomly selected doctors, and 197 acupuncturists. *Comp. Ther. Med.*, **4,** 8–13.

Noumi, T., Yamauchi, Y., Kamimura, K. *et al.* (1976). A broken acupuncture needle migrated into the spinal canal. *Nippon Iji Shinpo*, **4,** 799–803.

Oka, N., Kanemaru, K., Akiguchi, I. *et al.* (1986). Cervical adhesive arachnoiditis as a complication of acupuncture. *Rinsho Shineigaku*, **26,** 847–850.

Olusanya, O. and Mansuri, I. (1997). Pneumothorax following acupuncture. *J. Am. Board Fam. Pract.*, **10,** 296–297.

Peuker, E. T. and Filler, T. J. (1997a). Forensische Aspekte der Akupunktur. *Ärztezeitsch. Naturheilv.*, **38,** 833–842.

Peuker, E. T. and Filler, T. J. (1997b). The need for practical courses in anatomy for acupuncturists. *FACT*, **4,** 194.

Pierik, M. G. (1982). Fatal staphylococcal septicemia following acupuncture: Report of two cases. *R. I. Med. J.*, **65,** 251–253.

Rajanna, P. (1983). Hypotension following stimulation of acupuncture point fengchi (GB 20). *J. R. Coll. Gen. Pract.*, **303,** 606–607.

Rampes, H. (1998). Adverse reactions to acupuncture. In: *Medical Acupuncture: A Western Scientific Approach* (J. Filshie and A. White, eds), pp. 375–387. Edinburgh: Churchill Livingstone.

Rampes, H. and James, R. (1995). Complications of acupuncture. *Acupunct. Med.*, **13,** 26–33.

Redfearn, T. (1991). Oh, what a surprise! *Acupunct. Med.*, **9,** 2–3.

Ritter, H. G. and Tarala, R. (1978). Pneumothorax after acupuncture. *Br. Med. J.*, **277,** 602–603.

Rogers, P. A. M. (1981). Serious complications of acupuncture: or acupuncture abuses? *Am. J. Acupunct.*, **9,** 347–351.

Romaguera, C. and Grimalt, F. (1979). Nickel dermatitis from acupuncture needles. *Contact Dermatitis*, **5,** 195.

Romaguera, C. and Grimalt, F. (1981). Contact dermatitis from a permanent acupuncture needle. *Contact Dermatitis*, **7,** 156–157.

Roy, J. B. (1974). Acupuncture needle in bladder. *Urology*, **4,** 584.

Ruchkin, J. N. (1987). Auriculo-electroacupuncture in rheumatoid arthritis (a double blind study). *Ter. Arkh.*, **59,** 26–30.

Saenz, L., Lee, H. and Mottram, M. (1978). Permanent acupuncture needles. *JAMA*, **240,** 1482–1483.

Sasaki, H., Abe, H., Iwasaki, Y. *et al.* (1984). Direct spinal cord and root injury caused by acupuncture. Report of 2 cases. *No Shinkei Geka*, **12,** 1219–1223.

Sato, M., Yamane, K., Ezima, M. *et al.* (1991). A case of transverse myelopathy caused by acupuncture. *Rinsho Shinkeigaku*, **31,** 717–719.

Savage-Jones, H. (1985). Auricular complications of acupuncture. *J. Laryngol. Otol.*, **99,** 1143–1145.

Scheel, O., Sundsfjord, A., Lunde, P. and Andersen, B. M. (1992). Endocarditis after acupuncture and injection treatment by a natural healer. *JAMA*, **267,** 56.

Schiff, A. F. (1965). A fatality due to acupuncture. *Med. Times (Lond.)*, **93,** 630–631.

Schlenker, G. and Huegel, A. (1976). Complications of acupuncture. *Dtsch. Med. Wochenschr.*, **101,** 241.

Schmid, E., Hortling, G. and Kammuller, H. (1984). Inoculation hepatitis caused by acupuncture. Clinical cases studied over a 9 year period. *Fortschr. Med.*, **102,** 862–865.

Schneider, L. B. and Salzberg, M. R. (1984). Bilateral pneumothorax following acupuncture. *Ann. Emerg. Med.*, **13,** 643.

Schnorrenberger, C. (1978). Akupunktur: Schmerzschwelle wird erhöht. *Selecta*, **3,** 165.

Schratter, M., Bijak, M., Nissel, H. *et al.* (1997). Foramen sternale: Kleine Anomalie - große Relevanz. *Fortschr. Röntgenstr.*, **166,** 69–71.

Shiraishi, S., Goto, I., Kuroiwa, Y. *et al.* (1979). Spinal cord injury as a complication of an acupuncture. *Neurology*, **29,** 1180–1182.

Slater, P .E., Ben-Ishai, P., Leventhal, A. *et al.* (1988). An acupuncture-associated outbreak of hepatitis B in Jerusalem. *Eur. J. Epidemiol.*, **4,** 322–325.

Smith, D. L., Walczyk, M. H. and Campbell, S. (1989). Acupuncture needle induced compartment syndrome. *West. J. Med.*, **144,** 478–479.

Smith, P. F. and Rauscher, C. R. (1974). Complication of acupuncture. *JAMA*, **229,** 1286.

Sobel, E., Huang, E. and Wieting, C. (1997). Drop foot as a complication of acupuncture injury and intragluteal injection. *J. Am. Podiatr. Med. Assoc.*, **87,** 52–59.

Sorensen, T. (1990). Auricular perichondritis caused by acupuncture therapy. *Ugeskr. Laeger.*, **152,** 752–753.

Southworth, S. R. and Hartwig, R. H. (1990). Foreign body in the median nerve: a complication of acupuncture. *J. Hand Surg. (Br.)*, **15B,** 111–112.

Stack, B. H. R. (1975). Pneumothorax associated with acupuncture. *Br. Med. J.*, **1,** 96.

Stark, P. (1985). Midline sternal foramen: CT demonstration. *J. Comput. Assist. Tomogr.*, **9,** 489–490.

Stryker, W. S., Gunn, R. A. and Francis, D. P. (1986). Outbreak of hepatitis B associated with acupuncture. *J. Fam. Pract.*, **22,** 155–158.

Takishima, T. (1983). Pneumothorax as a complication of acupuncture in the treatment of bronchial asthma. *Ann. Allergy*, **51,** 402–403.

Tanii, T., Kono, T., Katoh, J. *et al.* (1991). A case of prurigo pigmentosa considered to be contact allergy to chromium in an acupuncture needle. *Acta Derm. Venereol. (Stockh.)*, **71,** 66–67.

Tanita, Y., Kato, T., Hanada, K. and Tagami, H. (1985). Blue macules of localised argyria caused by implanted acupuncture needles. *Arch. Dermatol.*, **121,** 1550–1552.

Tomonaga, I., Miyazaki, M., Kondo, T. *et al.* (1984). Migration of the acupuncture needles into the cervical spinal cord. *Orthop. Traumatol. (Fukuoka)*, **32,** 123–125.

Trautermann, H. G. and Trautermann, H. (1981). Perichondritis der Ohrmuschel nach Akupunktur. *HNO*, **29,** 312–313.

Tsukerman, I. M. (1970). A rare case of carcinoma of the skin arising after acupuncture. *Vopr. Onkol.*, **16,** 88.

Tuke, J. (1979). Complication of acupuncture. *Br. Med. J.*, **2,** 1076.

Umeh, B. (1989). Moxibustion: respiratory complications. *Acupunct. Med.*, **6,** 61–62.

Umlauf, R. (1988). Analysis of the main results of the activity of the acupuncture department of faculty hospital. *Acupunct. Med.*, **5,** 16–18.

Valenta, L. and Hengesh, J. (1980). Pneumothorax caused by acupuncture. *Lancet*, **330,** 322.

Verma, S. K. and Khamesra, R. (1989). Recurrent fainting – an unusual reaction to acupuncture. *J. Assoc. Physicians India*, **37,** 600.

Vilke, G., Wulfert, E. (1997). Case reports of two patients with pneumothorax following acupuncture. *J. Emerg. Med.*, **15,** 155–157.

Vittecoq, D., Mettetal, J. F., Rouzioux, C. *et al.* (1989a). Acute HIV infection after acupuncture treatments. *N. Engl. J. Med.*, **320,** 250–251.

Vittecoq, D., Mettetal, J. F., Rouzioux, C. *et al.* (1989b). Unusual modes of HIV transmission. *N. Engl. J. Med.*, **321,** 1477.

Waldman, I. (1974). Pneumothorax from acupuncture. *N. Engl. J. Med.*, **290,** 633.

Warwick-Brown, N. P. and Richards, A. E. S. (1986). Perichondritis of the ear following acupuncture. *J. Laryngol. Otol.*, **100,** 1177–1179.

Wex, P. and Weig, J. (1978). Spontanpneumothorax – Ätiologie – Behandlungsplan und Ergebnisse. *Prax. Pneumol.*, **32,** 593–597.

White, A., Hayhoe, S. and Ernst, E. (1997). Survey of adverse events following acupuncture. *Acupunct. Med.*, **15,** 67–70.

Willms, D. (1991). Possible complications of acupuncture. *West. J. Med.*, **154,** 736–737.

Wright, R. S., Kupperman, J. L. and Liebhaber, M. L. (1991). Bilateral tension pneumothoraces after acupuncture. *West. J. Med.*, **154,** 102–103.

Yamaguchi, S., Kyakuno, M. and Osafune, M. (1989). Foreign body in the kidney: a case report and a review of the Japanese literature. *Hinyokika Kiyo*, **35,** 665–669.

Yin, Y. C. (1937). Wire needle in the abdominal cavity: an accident in acupuncture. *Chin. Med. J.*, **52,** 107–108.

Yuzawa, M., Hara, Y., Kobayashi, Y. *et al.* (1991). Foreign body stone of the ureter as a complication of acupuncture: report of a case. *Hinyokika Kiyo*, **37,** 1323–1327.

Conclusion

Edzard Ernst and Adrian White

The introduction to this book described the increasing integration of acupuncture into health care services in the west. Health care should meet stringent criteria of efficacy, safety and cost, in order to provide optimal benefit for patients, at minimal risk. This book was aimed at summarizing the relevant evidence regarding acupuncture in an impartial way. The conclusions are neither simple nor uniform.

The first requirement is for evidence of efficacy. The only compelling evidence that acupuncture is efficacious is for the treatment of the following conditions:

1. Back pain: which lends support to its widespread use in pain clinics for this indication.
2. Nausea: although the clinical impact of this remains uncertain until it is widely available.
3. Dental pain: efficacy shown in experimental conditions may not be sufficiently powerful to be useful clinically.

Systematic reviews of the evidence do not support the efficacy of acupuncture in other conditions for which it is frequently used: the evidence in neck pain, headache and asthma is insufficient, and in osteoarthritis is highly contradictory. The evidence for an effect in recovery from stroke is promising but far from convincing. Acupuncture seems to have no specific effect on smoking cessation or dieting. Thus, at present, we cannot say with certainty that acupuncture is truly useful in a large range of clinical conditions.

Second, acupuncture should be shown to be safe. Adverse effects of acupuncture, some of them life threatening, are well documented. However, far too little is known of their incidence and further necessary research is underway to answer the open questions. All we can state at present is that acupuncture is not free of risks. These may be rarities. In order to take this notion beyond the level of speculation we need data rather than beliefs.

Third, acupuncture should be demonstrated to be at least as cheap as other available therapies for individual conditions. The economic evaluation of acupuncture has not been addressed in this book, because no reliable studies have yet been performed. However, some trials have suggested that considerable savings may be expected, for example in osteoarthritis of the knee and stroke (White, 1996). Certainly, acupuncture needles are not expensive (although acupuncturists may prove to be!). In the competition for scarce resources, proper cost-effectiveness and cost–benefit analyses of acupuncture will be required.

Acupuncture: popular and efficacious?

One may well ask why acupuncture is so popular when the evidence of its effectiveness is so fragmentary. There are well-known reasons for the rise in usage of complementary medicine in general (Furnham, 1996; Astin, 1998). These include both the negative aspects of conventional treatment (lack of effectiveness for chronic conditions, fear of side-effects, lack of practitioner time) and the positive aspects of complementary medicine (perceived as more holistic, and considered natural therefore safe).

There are additional reasons to explain the rise in acupuncture in particular. Acupuncture has many positive attractions for patients: it is clearly out of the ordinary, it involves Oriental mystique, and (importantly) offers time with the therapist. It is perceived as holistic, it involves touch and personal dedication, and it produces definite sensations. The reader will readily appreciate that these are also features that render one placebo more effective than another! Whatever else is discovered about acupuncture, it appears to be a powerful, even a perfect, placebo.

Acupuncture is also popular with practitioners. Those who practise traditional Chinese acupuncture (TCA) are captivated by its ancient Oriental origins and complex philosophy. Kaptchuk and Birch (see Chapter 1) have shown how a traditional diagnosis involves co-ordinating information about every aspect of the patient's symptoms, tastes and preferences, including, for example, their choice in food. In many ways, this appears to be largely an art, and TCA may epitomize the debate between the role of art and science in medicine. While accepting that the philosophical approach of TCA is attractive to both patients and practitioners, modern health care requires more: for one thing, it insists that any therapeutic approach is constantly modified and updated in response to new research evidence (see Chapter 2). The traditional approach to acupuncture should not be rejected simply on the grounds that its theory appears to be contrary to current scientific knowledge. However, practitioners of TCA should seek evidence of efficacy from rigorous trials in the same way as western acupuncture or any other therapy.

The debate whether medicine is an art or a science is, in our view, not very productive. Good medicine, we feel, should encompass the art and work towards perfecting the science. Art and science are not alternatives, they are truly complementary: one without the other constitutes medicine that is less than optimal.

The rapid growth of acupuncture is partly a result of its acceptance within orthodox medicine in many countries, particularly for pain control and rehabilitation medicine. This followed the discovery of the opioid peptides, or 'endorphins', in the 1970s. The endorphins provided a mechanism that could explain acupuncture, which became instantly respectable. In fact, the evidence reviewed in Chapter 3 shows that opioid peptides have a rather small role to play, at least in acupuncture's effect on acute experimental pain. Other mechanisms have been investigated, including the release of calcitonin gene-related peptide (CGRP) and reduced sympathetic tone (see Chapter 4), but are yet to be incontrovertibly proven. The realization that the mechanism is fundamentally neurological also provided a basis for a new approach to the practice of acupuncture, independent of traditional theories, viz the trigger point and segmental techniques (see Chapter 2).

However, acupuncture should not be integrated into health care provision for the reasons that it is philosophically attractive or because its mechanisms are plausible. Patients' interests demand that it be demonstrated how effective and safe it is for defined conditions.

Seeking evidence

There is no doubt that designing and performing rigorous clinical trials in acupuncture brings particular methodological problems, which have been discussed in Chapter 2. There are indications that these problems are at last being solved. We are therefore hopeful that progress in seeking evidence will now be rapid.

Subject-blinding requires that control groups should be treated with a procedure that they find indistinguishable from genuine acupuncture. A series of investigations is planned in the USA into what constitutes an acceptable sham procedure (B. M. Berman, personal communication). A strong candidate must be the use of a new sham needle in which the needle shaft telescopes into the handle, giving the impression that it is advancing through the tissues (Streitberger and Kleinhenz, 1998). This novelty from Germany is the most promising advance for some time, although problems still remain.

Exactly as when testing new drugs, trials of acupuncture need to be planned by experts in trial methodology, statistics, etc. If there is a difference from conventional trials, acupuncture trials are more complex and therefore require more thorough planning than other clinical studies. For example, control interventions cannot necessarily be assumed to be totally without physiological effect; thus, large sample sizes are required in order to show small differences in clinical trials.

The evidence on mechanisms in Chapters 3 and 4 has suggested one area of concern that is still unresolved. It appears that the response of any individual to acupuncture can vary from nil to a maximum. The factors behind this variability are not understood. There is some evidence that psychological 'preparedness' may be crucial in predicting a response. Filshie and Cummings (see Chapter 2) pointed out that placebo and acupuncture may each stimulate, at least in part, the same neurophysiological system, i.e. the opioid peptides.

When the efficacy of acupuncture is being examined in clinical trials, it should be applied in a manner that is accepted by a wide section of the profession to be adequate for the indication being investigated. Given two main underlying theoretical approaches, it seems inevitable that trials will have to be duplicated. Perhaps individual schools will be encouraged to provide rigorous evidence of the success of their approach.

Promising conditions for trials can be selected from evidence of cohort studies, and from the conditions listed in Chapter 5 for which the evidence is contradictory or inconclusive.

Unravelling the effects of acupuncture from those of placebo will be a fascinating, challenging but necessary task.

Possible outcomes of further research

The current evidence of the efficacy of acupuncture could be compatible with several eventual conclusions, each with important consequences for the integration of this therapy within health services, for the training of practitioners and for further research. Different outcomes are, of course, likely in different conditions.

Outcome 1

In the event (rather unlikely, based on current evidence) that acupuncture proves to do more harm than good, then it should be abandoned. Most harm associated with acupuncture appears to be a result of poor practice. Therefore, it should be avoidable through greater attention to training standards.

Outcome 2

Research may establish beyond reasonable doubt that acupuncture is shown to have the same effect as sham acupuncture, for a particular condition. Both could still be useful for their non-specific effects. Then the safest effective form of acupuncture should be administered, whether it involves needling or not. Practitioners should be trained in effective placebo therapy rather than acupuncture points. Research should investigate what constitutes effective placebo therapy and how this can be optimized, both for acupuncture and for other forms of treatment.

Outcome 3

Traditional Chinese acupuncture could prove to be superior to western medical acupuncture (and to sham) for a particular condition. In this case, TCA should be integrated into health care, and should be the method taught in acupuncture colleges. Research should address the question of optimizing methods of diagnosis and treatment, as well as exploring the underlying mechanisms.

Outcome 4

Western acupuncture could prove superior to TCA (and to sham) for a particular condition. In this case, acupuncture should be practised within a western medical context. Teaching should concentrate on conventional diagnostic methods and treatment approaches. Research should optimize the clinical technique and further explore underlying mechanisms. TCA would become a subject for sociologists and medical historians to study.

Clearly, the evidence presented in this book is sufficiently in favour of acupuncture to amply justify further rigorously designed and well-performed investigations. Indeed, there is a responsibility to answer the questions of efficacy, safety and cost in the best interests of patients.

References

Astin, J. A. (1998). Why patients use alternative medicine: results of a national study. *JAMA*, **279**, 1548–1553.

Furnham, A. (1996). Why do people choose and use complementary therapies? In *Complementary Medicine: An Objective Appraisal* (E. Ernst, ed.), pp. 71–88. Oxford: Butterworth-Heinemann.

Streitberger, K. and Kleinhenz, J. (1998). Introducing a placebo needle into acupuncture research. *Lancet*, **352**, 364–365.

White, A. R. (1996). Do complementary therapies offer value for money? In *Complementary Medicine: An Objective Appraisal* (E. Ernst, ed.), pp. 89–105. Oxford: Butterworth-Heinemann.

Index

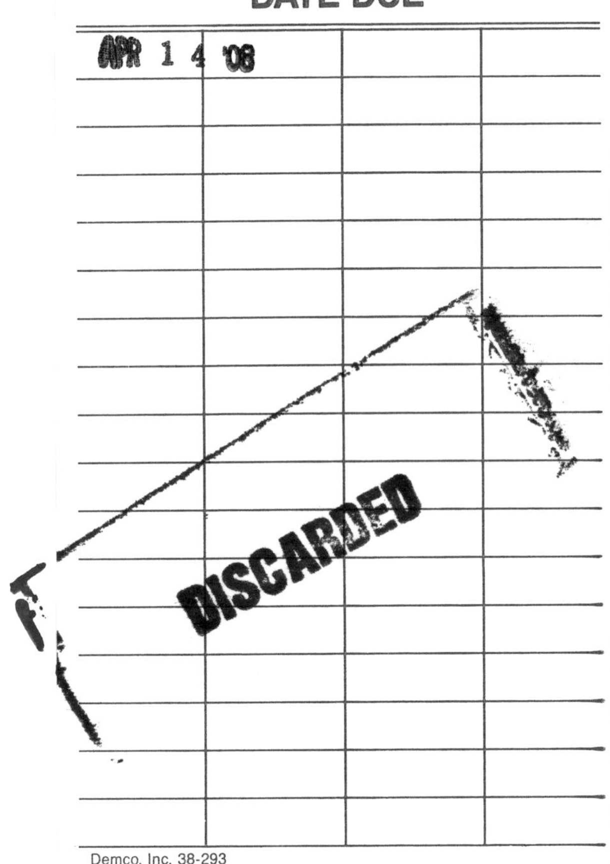